Meet the FRIENDLIES!

Getting to Know Your GOOD BACTERIA

Written by
Dr. Philippa Norman

Illustrated by Marcia Adams Ho

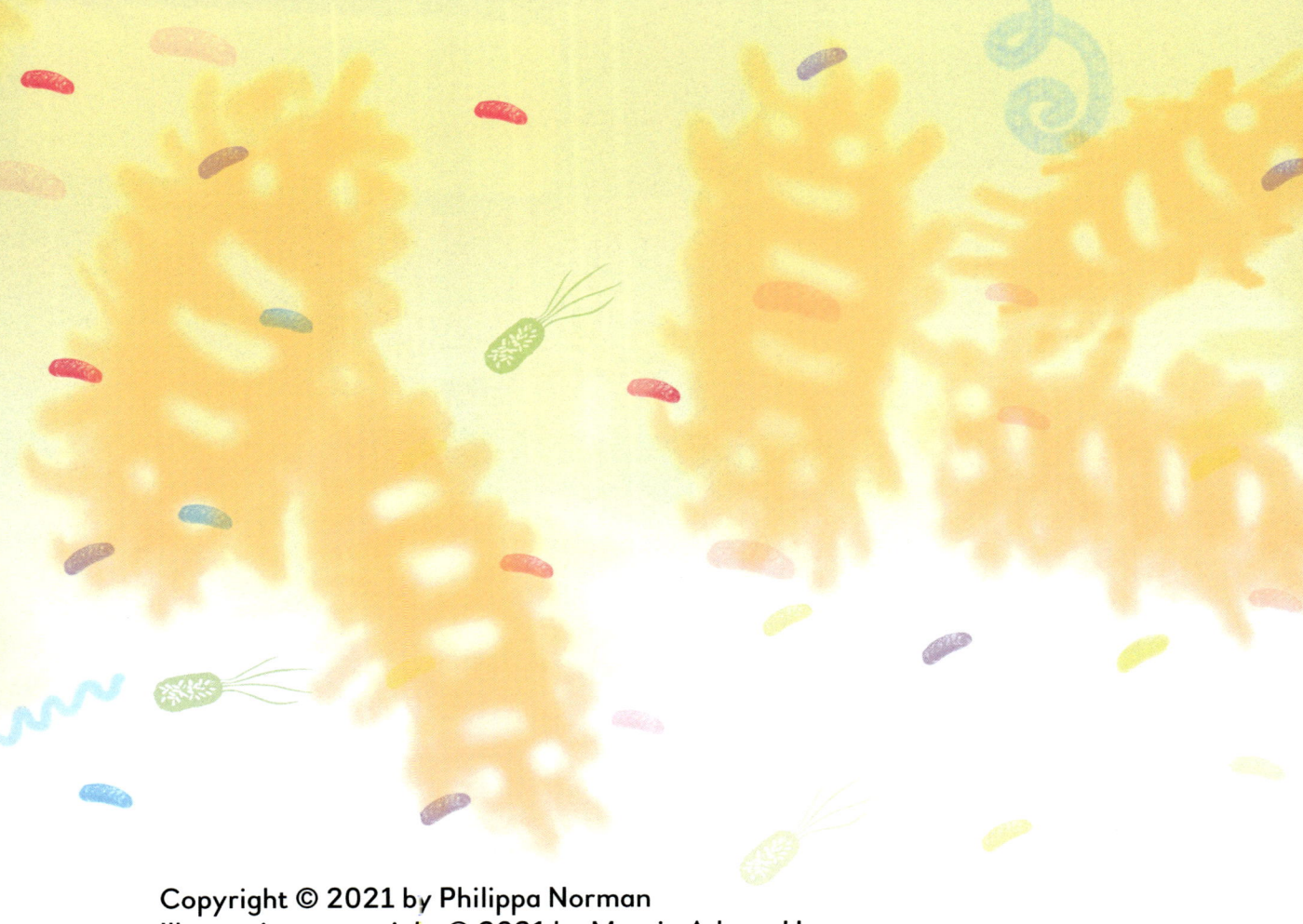

Copyright © 2021 by Philippa Norman
Illustrations copyright © 2021 by Marcia Adams Ho
All rights reserved.

No portion of this book may be reproduced — mechanically, electronically, or by any other means, including photocopying — without written permission of the publisher. Library of Congress Cataloging in Publication Data can be obtained from the Library of Congress.

First Edition
ISBN: 978-1-892742-05-6
Oak Park, Illinois

Disclaimer:
This book is not intended to substitute for health advice or medical care.

WWW.PHILIPPANORMANMD.COM

Table of Contents

PART 1
Meeting Your Friendlies **7**

PART 2
How to Grow Your Friendly Family **41**

PART 3
Glossary **59**

NOTE: Words in orange can be found in the glossary.

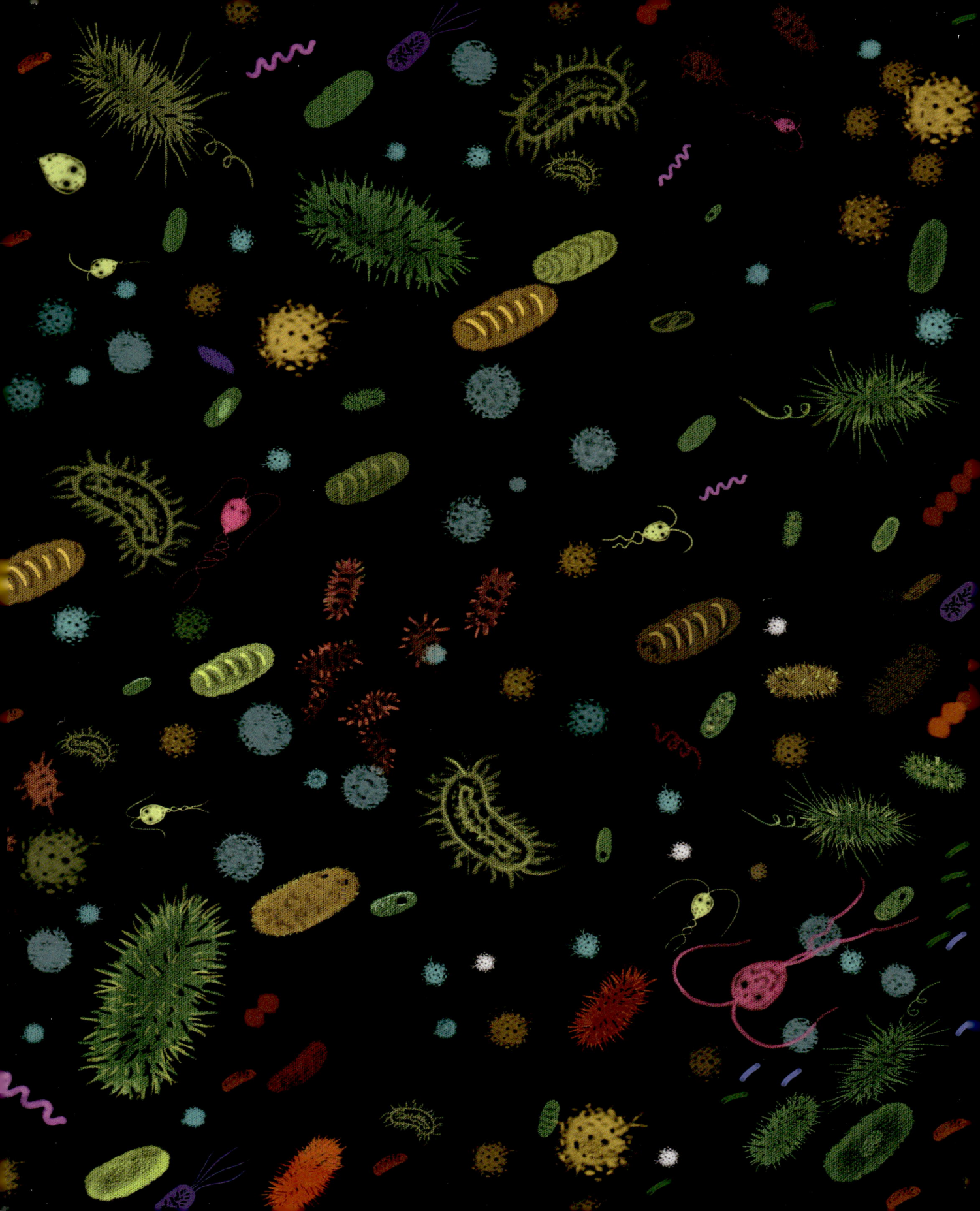

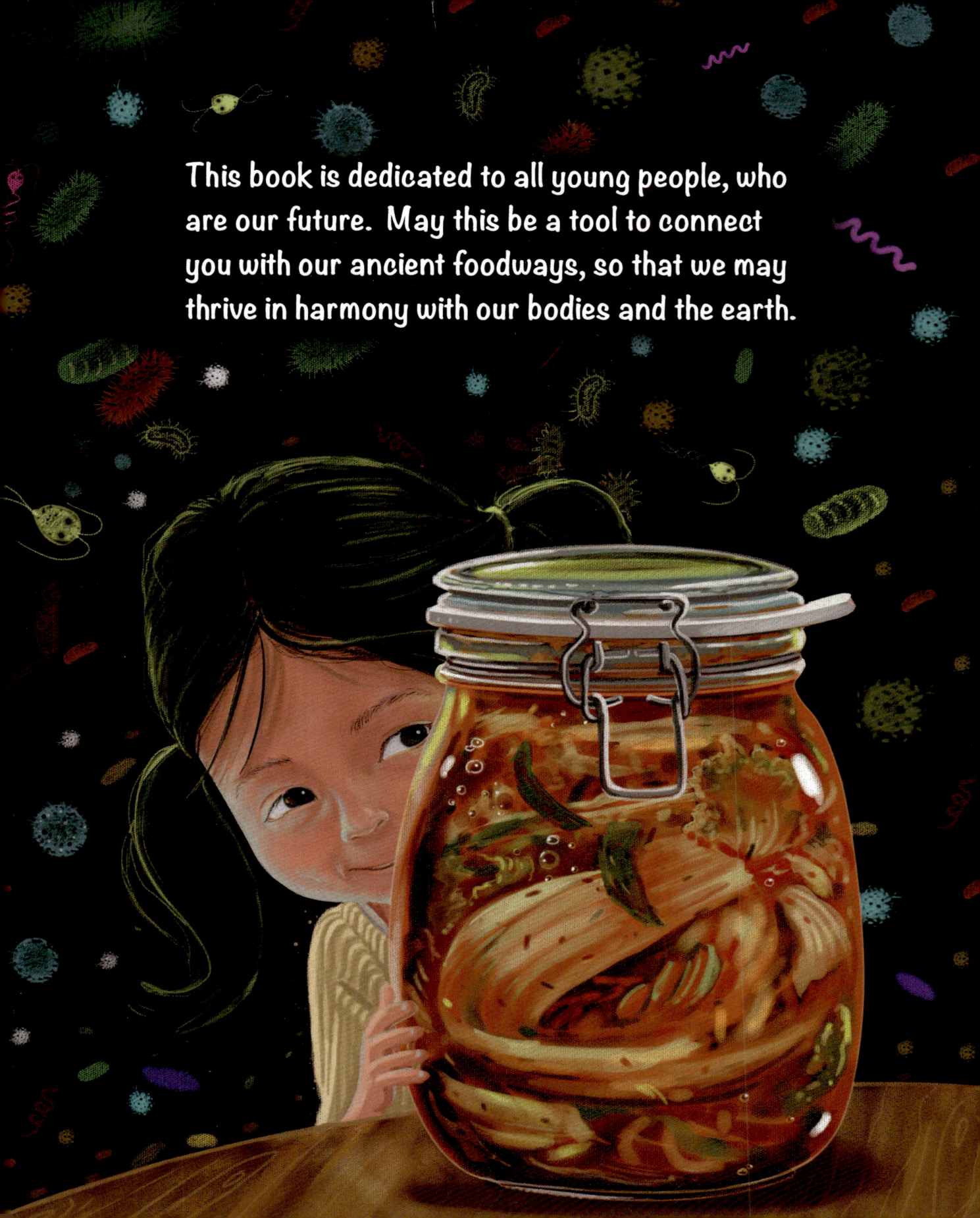

This book is dedicated to all young people, who are our future. May this be a tool to connect you with our ancient foodways, so that we may thrive in harmony with our bodies and the earth.

You have billions of friends.

They live with you every day.

They are called **bacteria**.

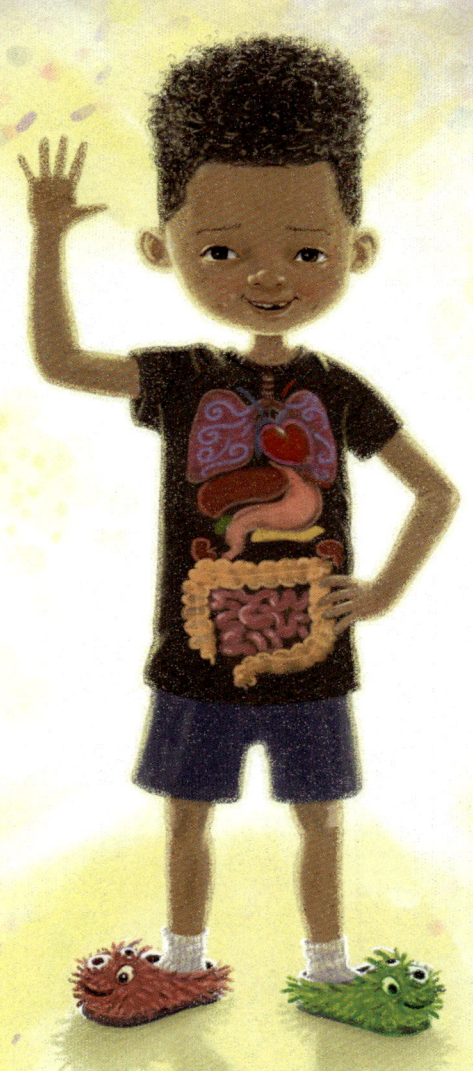

They are living things

So small, one thousand of them can live on this dot .

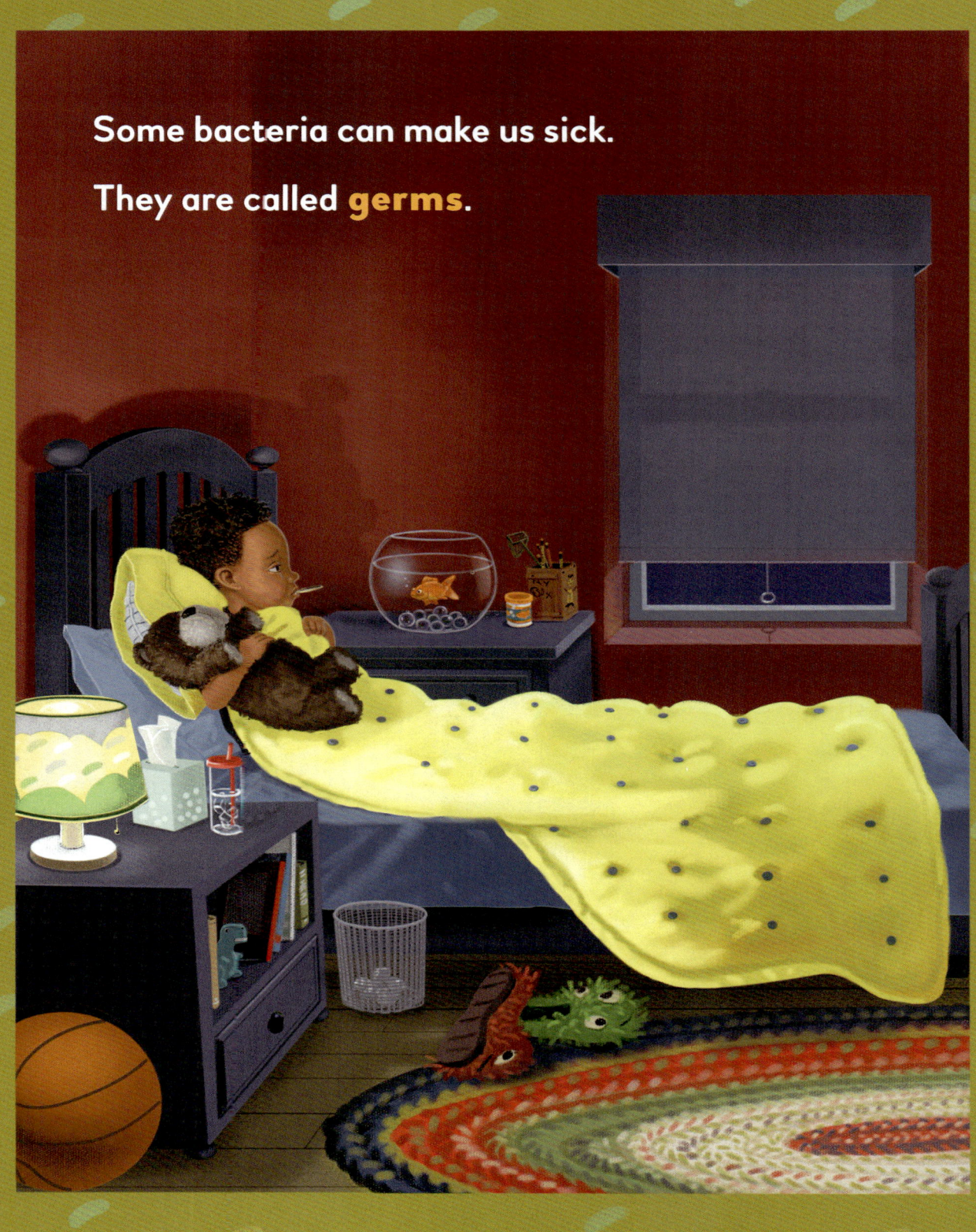

Some bacteria can make us sick.

They are called **germs**.

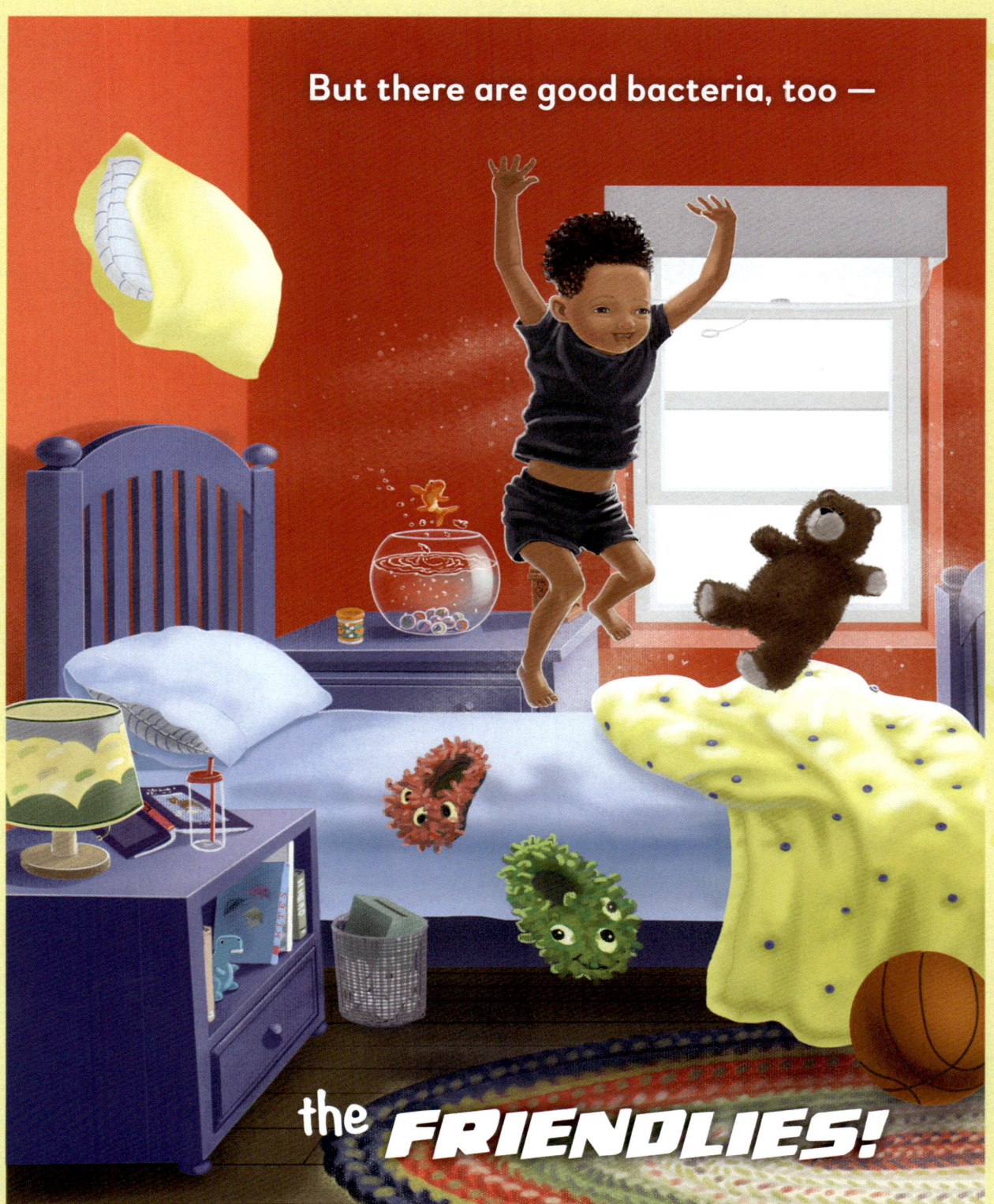

Friendlies have been on the Earth for over 4 billion years.

They live in many different environments, or habitats in nature.

They adapt to their surroundings.

Some float in the moisture of clouds, while others live in dry sand.

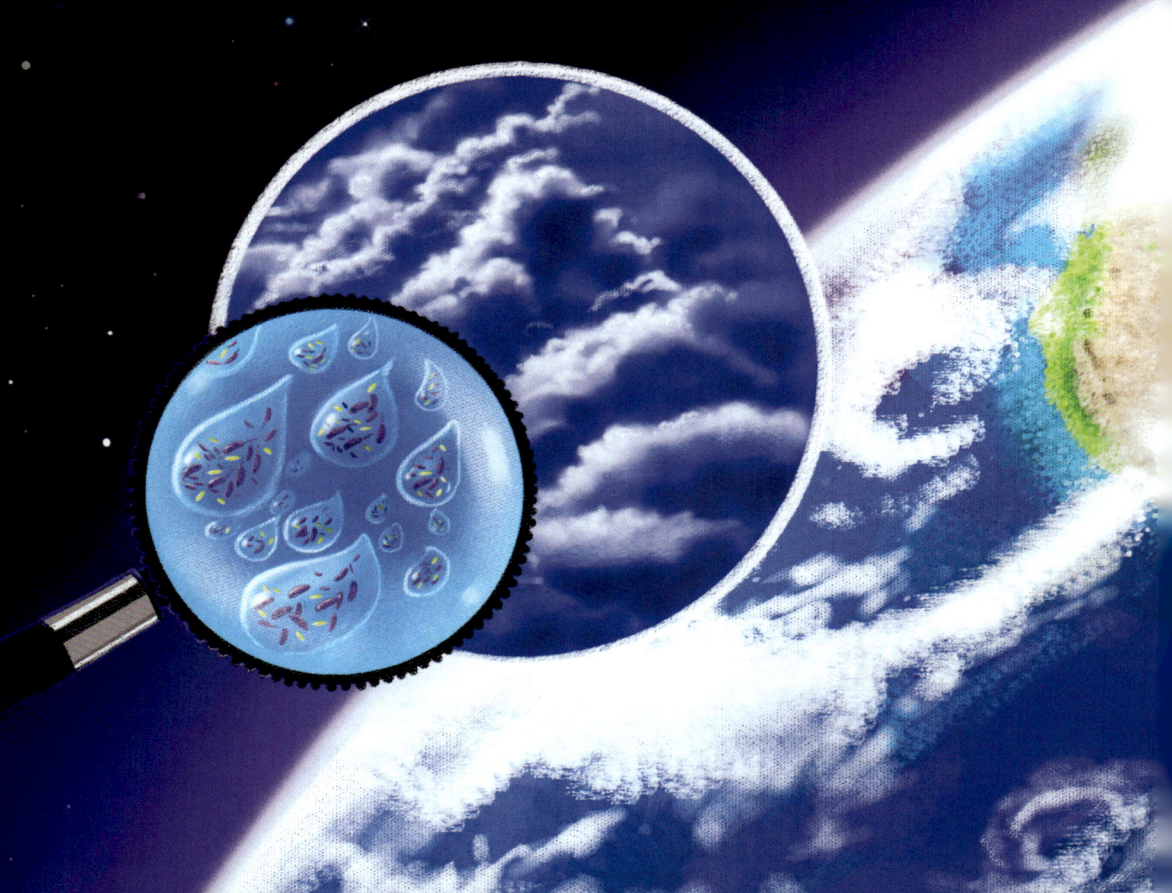

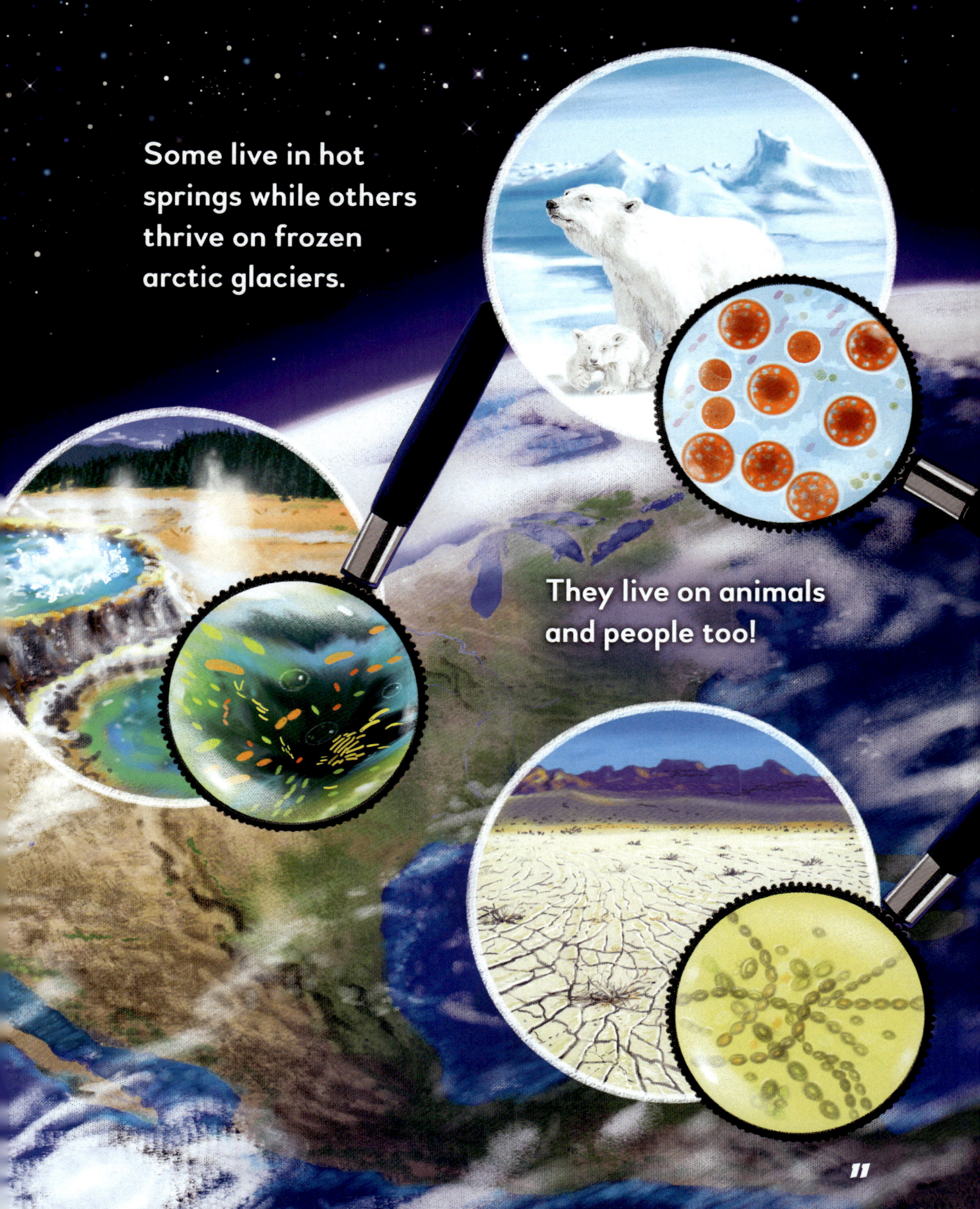

Some live in hot springs while others thrive on frozen arctic glaciers.

They live on animals and people too!

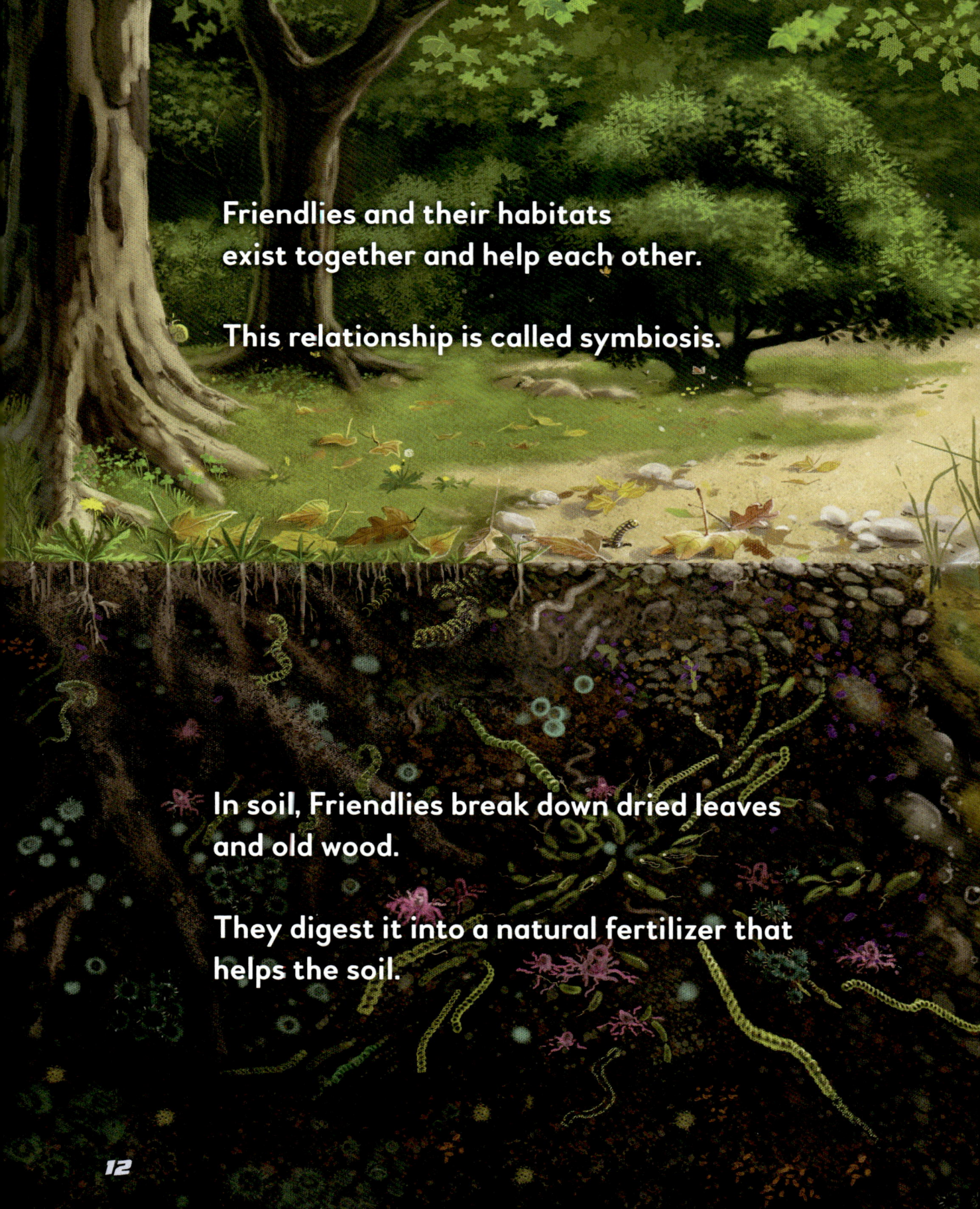

Friendlies and their habitats exist together and help each other.

This relationship is called symbiosis.

In soil, Friendlies break down dried leaves and old wood.

They digest it into a natural fertilizer that helps the soil.

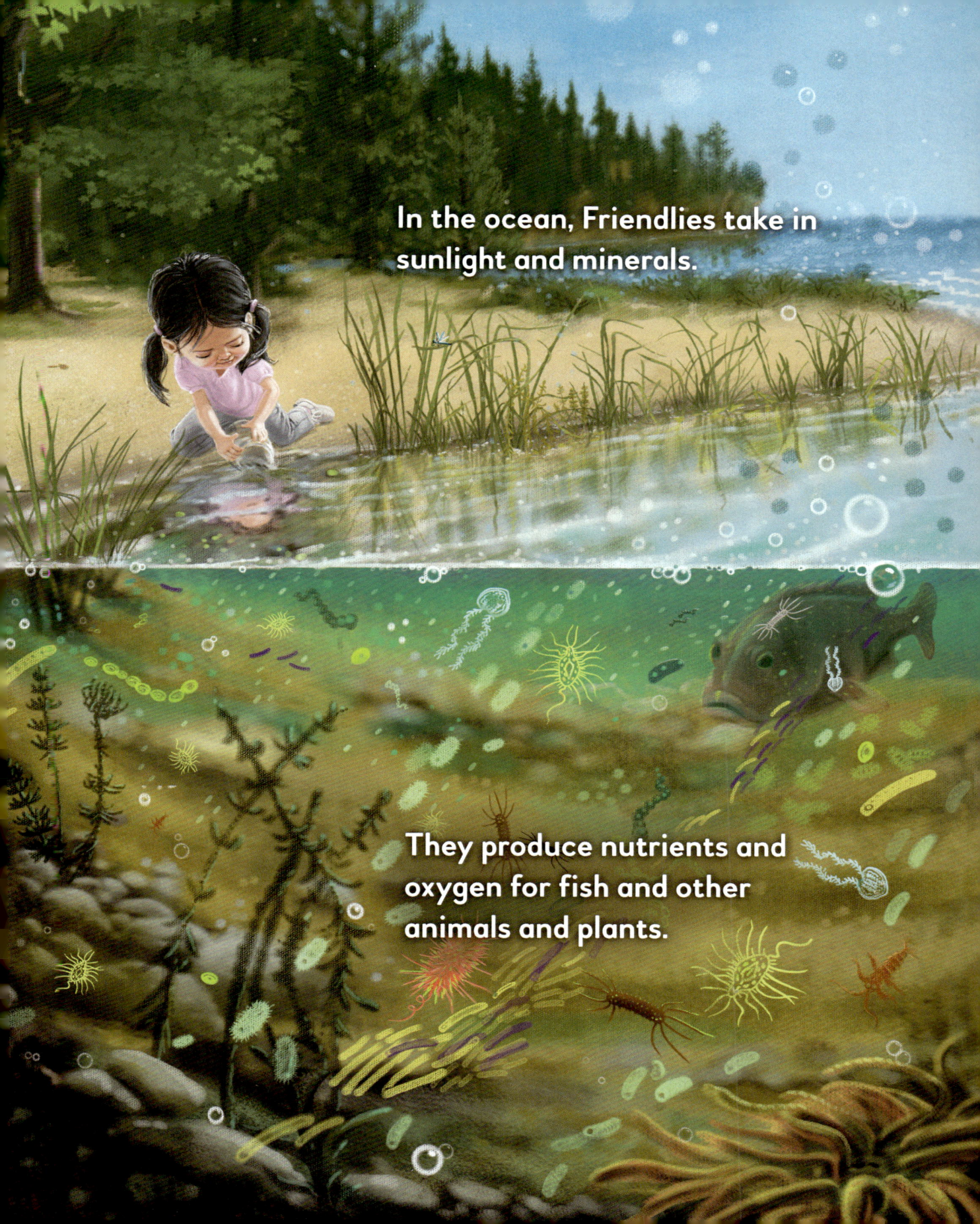

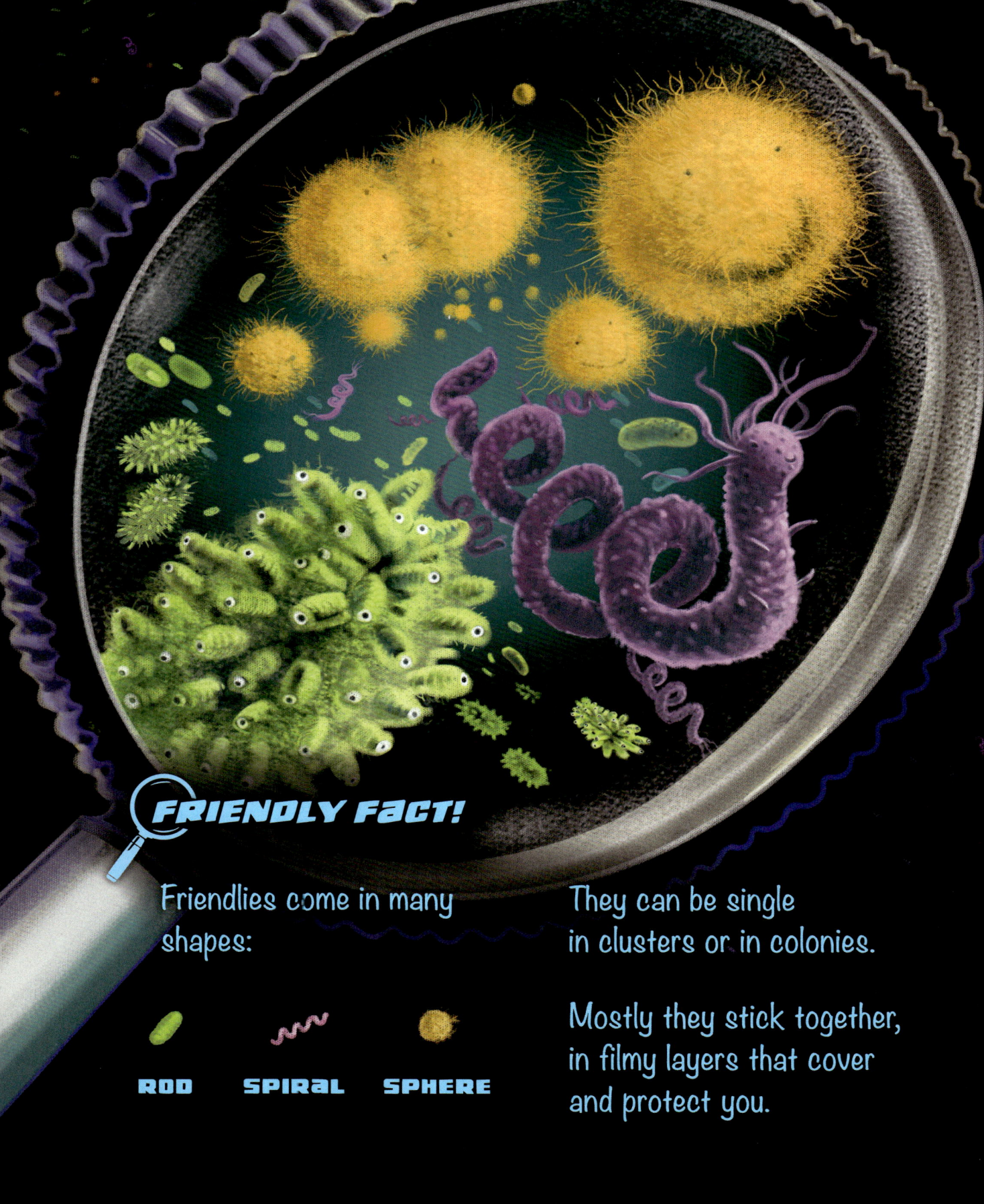

FRIENDLY FACT!

Friendlies come in many shapes:

ROD **SPIRAL** **SPHERE**

They can be single in clusters or in colonies.

Mostly they stick together, in filmy layers that cover and protect you.

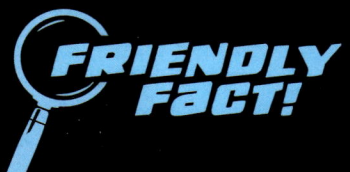

How did you get your Friendlies?

They coated you when you were born.

They settled on you from the breeze.

They come from the food you eat, people and pets too!

Friendlies live on and inside of you. They are part of the **immune system**.

You are a habitat for Friendlies!

The creases of your nose and ears have oil glands that make sebum.

Friendlies break down the sebum making a protective layer of gentle acid for your skin.

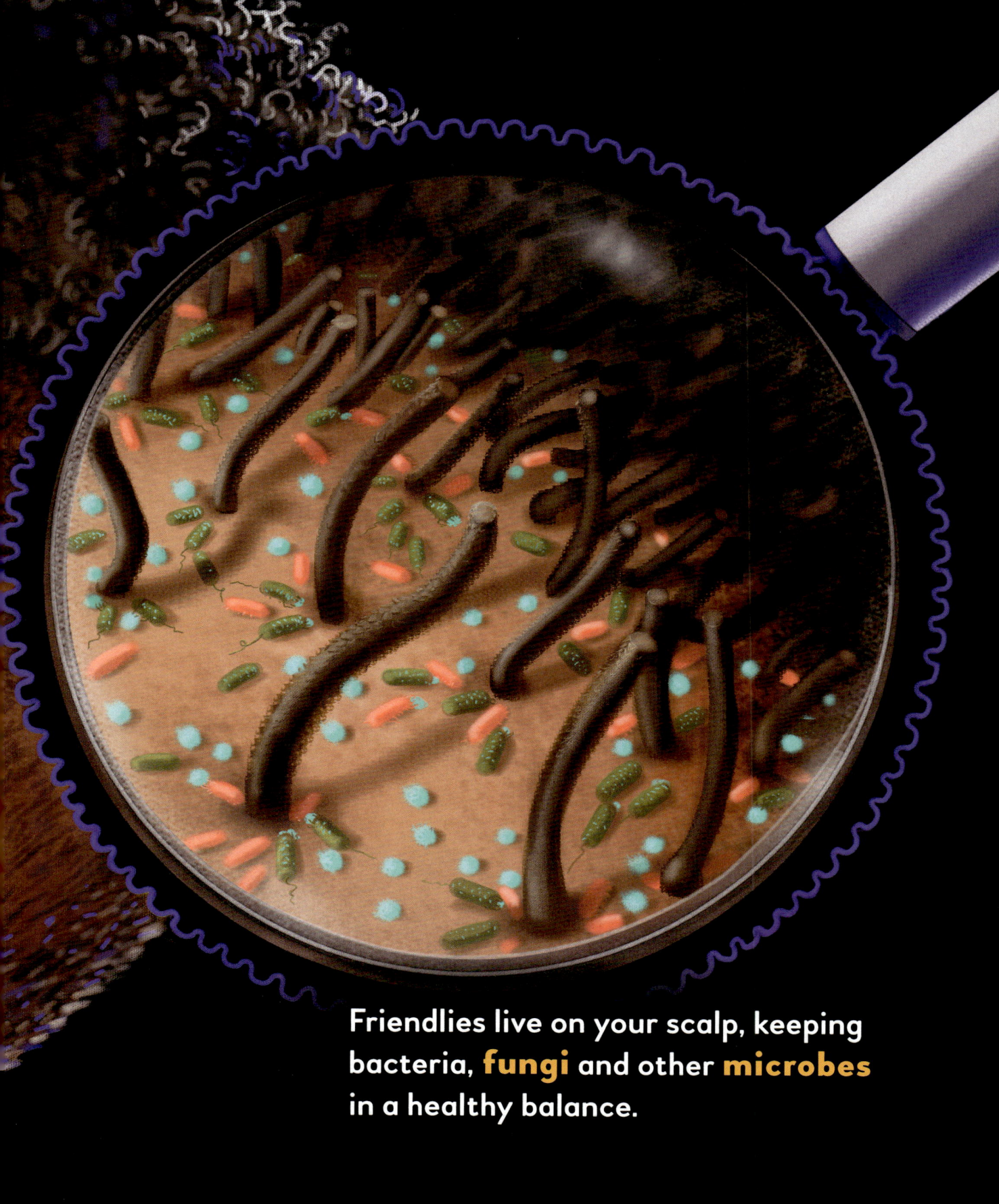

Friendlies live on your scalp, keeping bacteria, **fungi** and other **microbes** in a healthy balance.

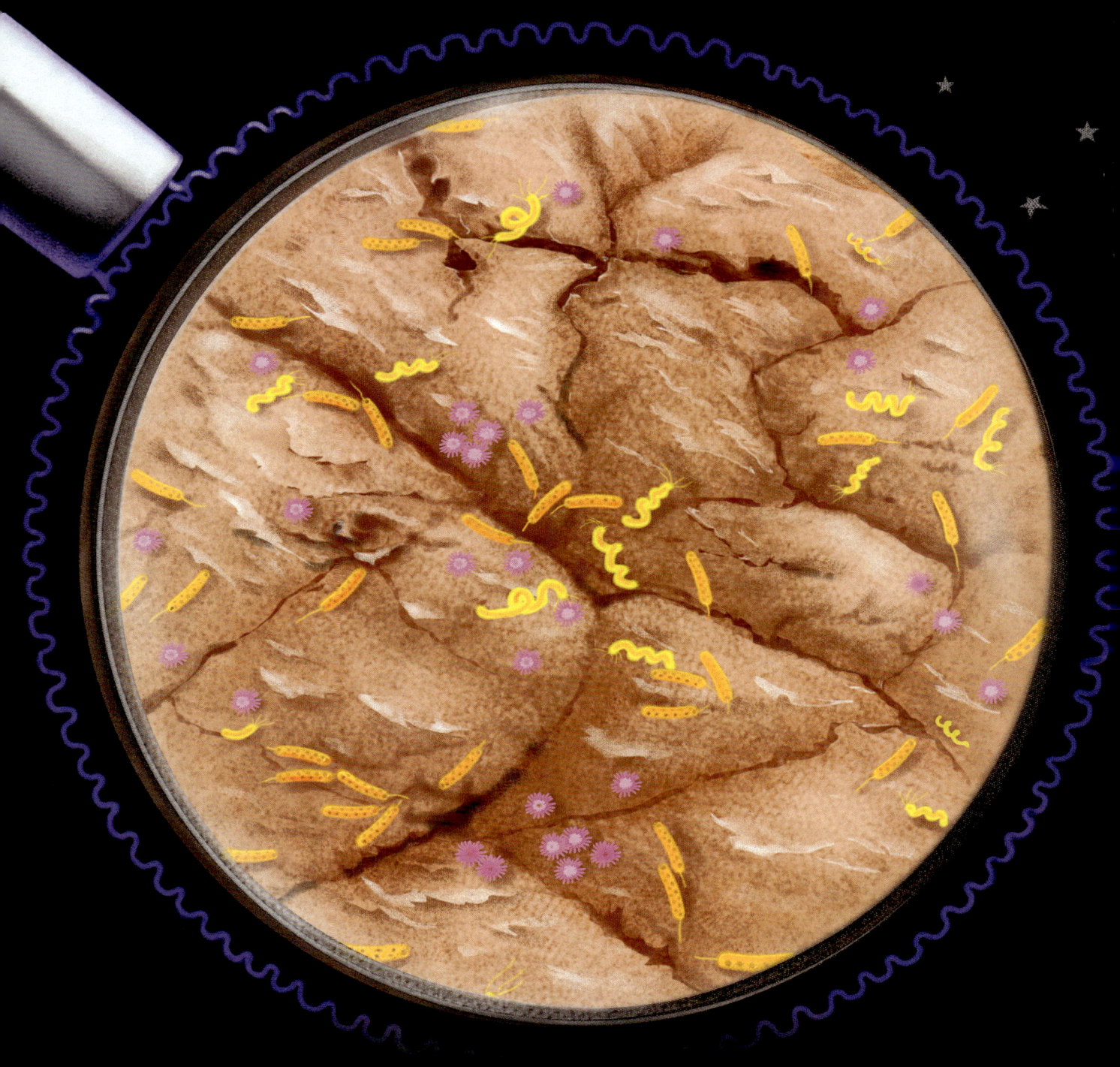

Friendlies adapt to each habitat of your body. Arms and legs are more like a dry desert, compared to the oily areas around the nose and ears.

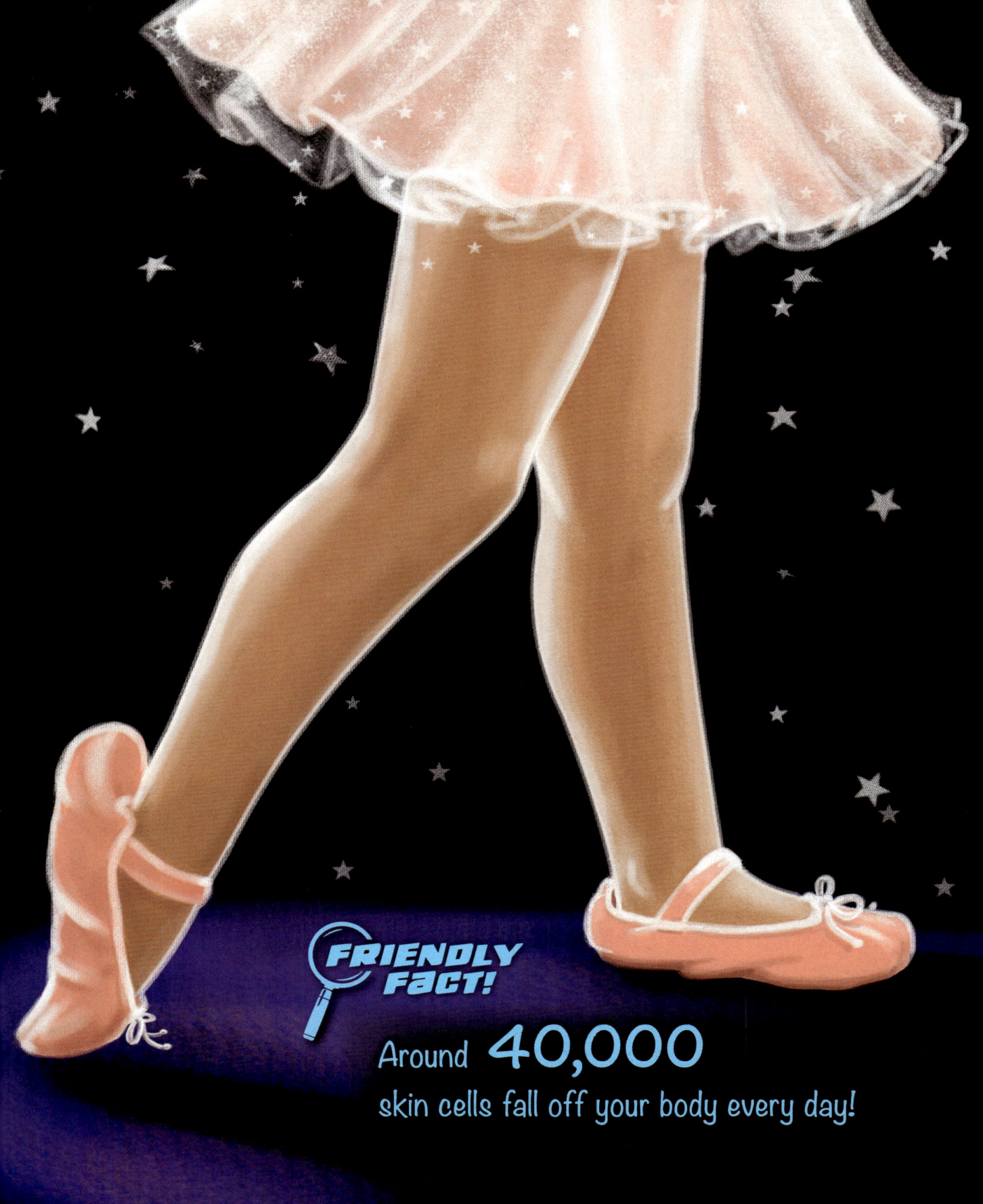

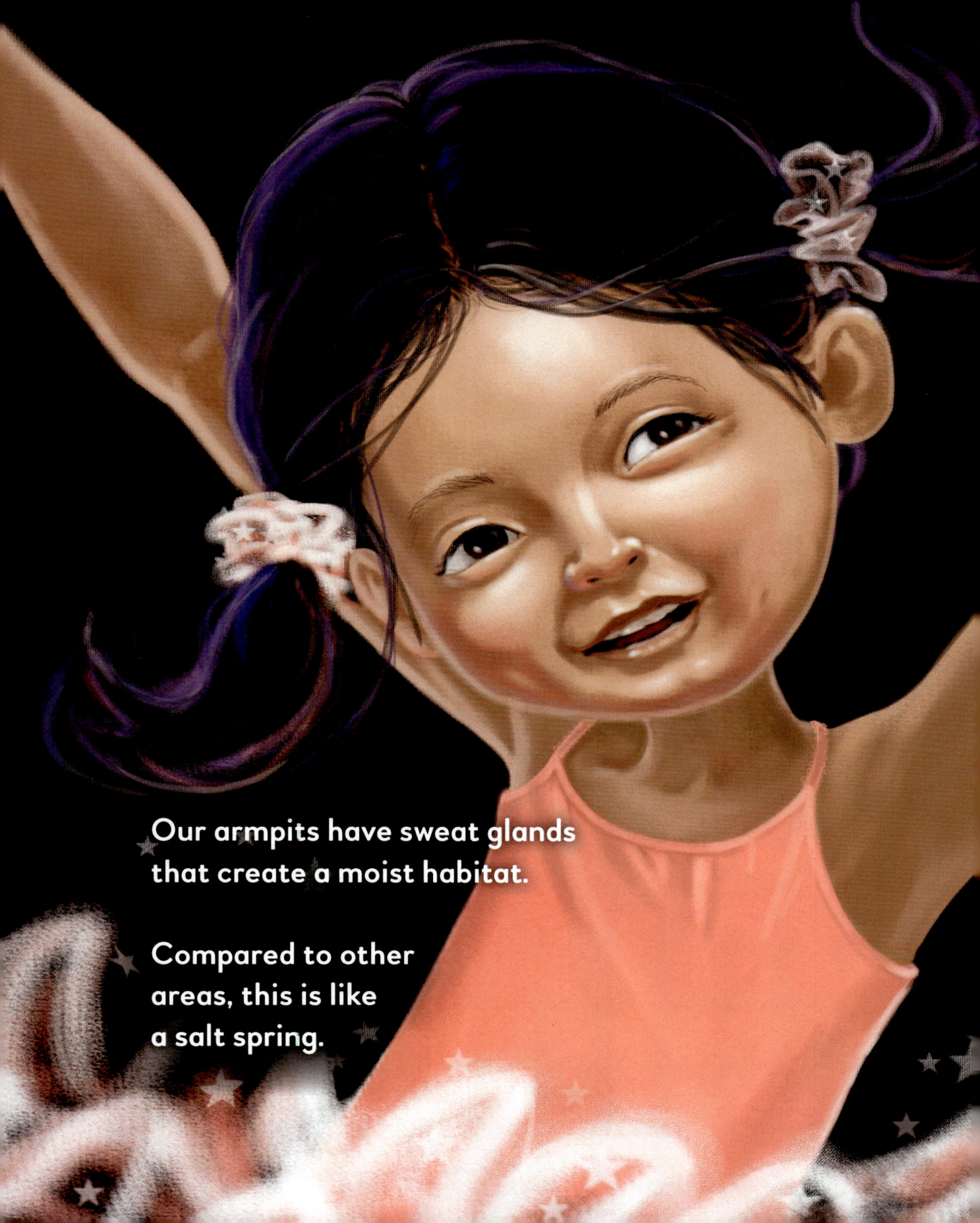

Our armpits have sweat glands that create a moist habitat.

Compared to other areas, this is like a salt spring.

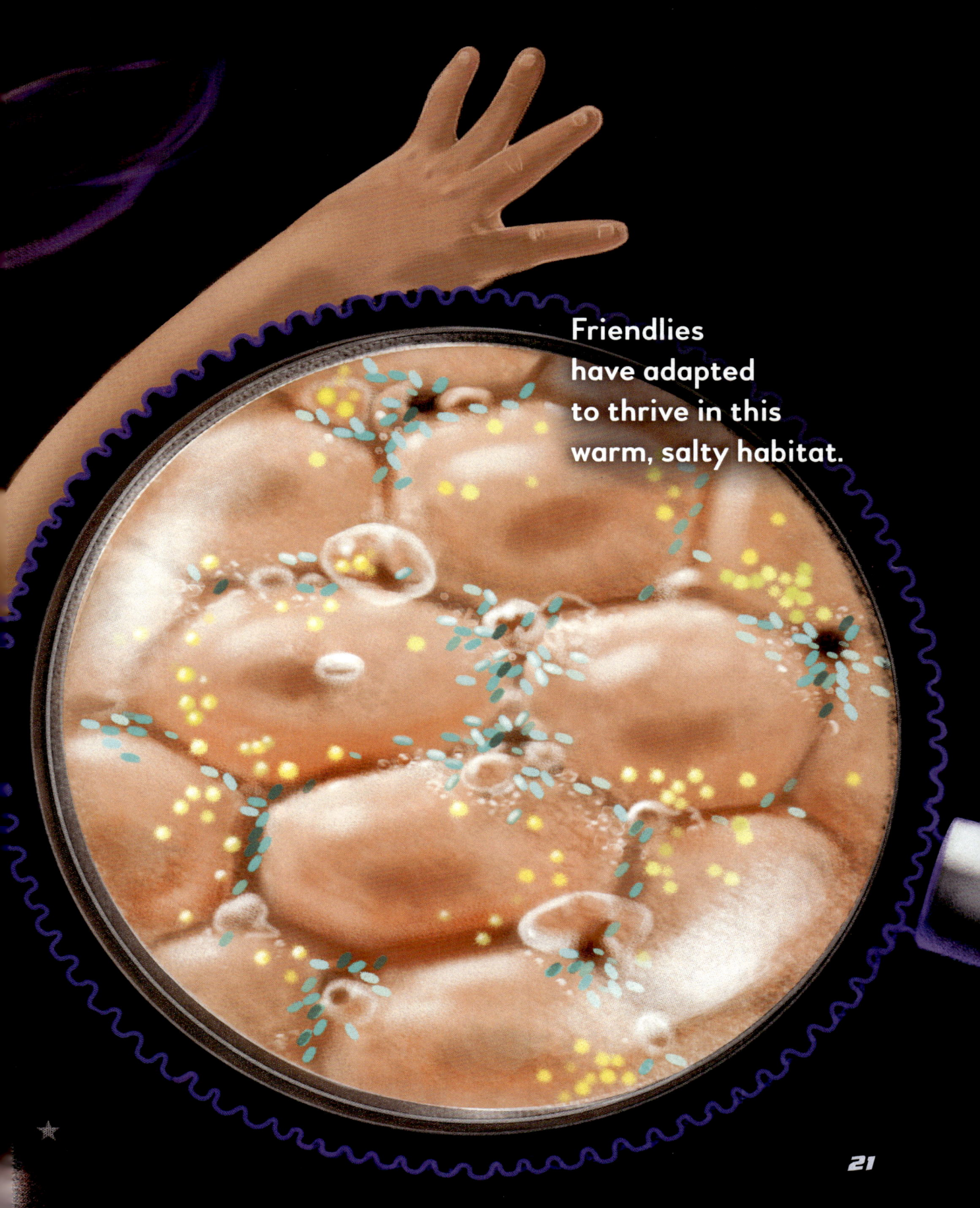

Friendlies have adapted to thrive in this warm, salty habitat.

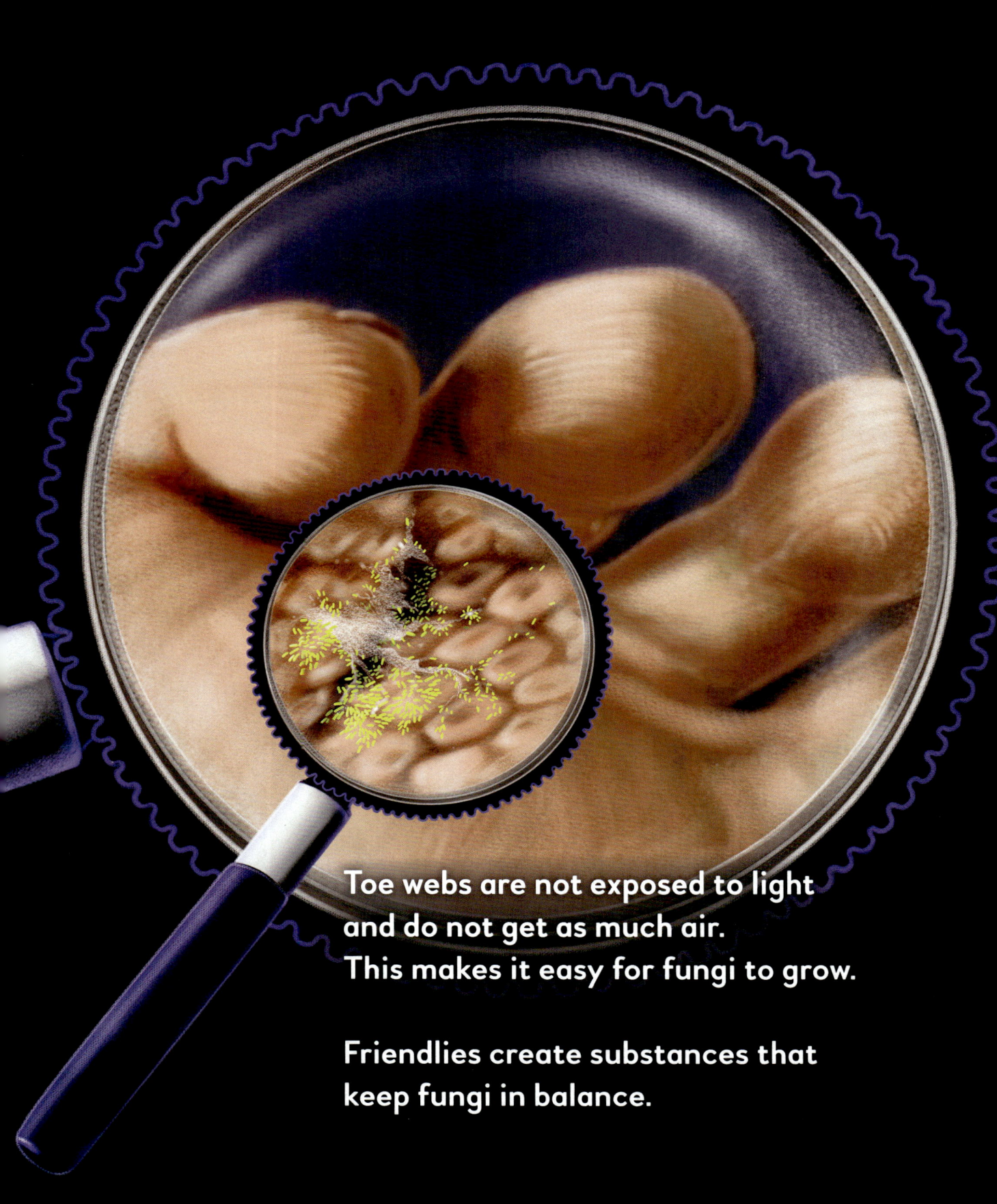

Toe webs are not exposed to light and do not get as much air.
This makes it easy for fungi to grow.

Friendlies create substances that keep fungi in balance.

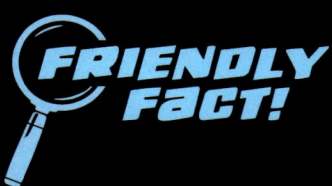

FRIENDLY FACT!

Keeping toes dry and clean helps prevent fungi from growing too much

(and helps keep Friendlies strong)

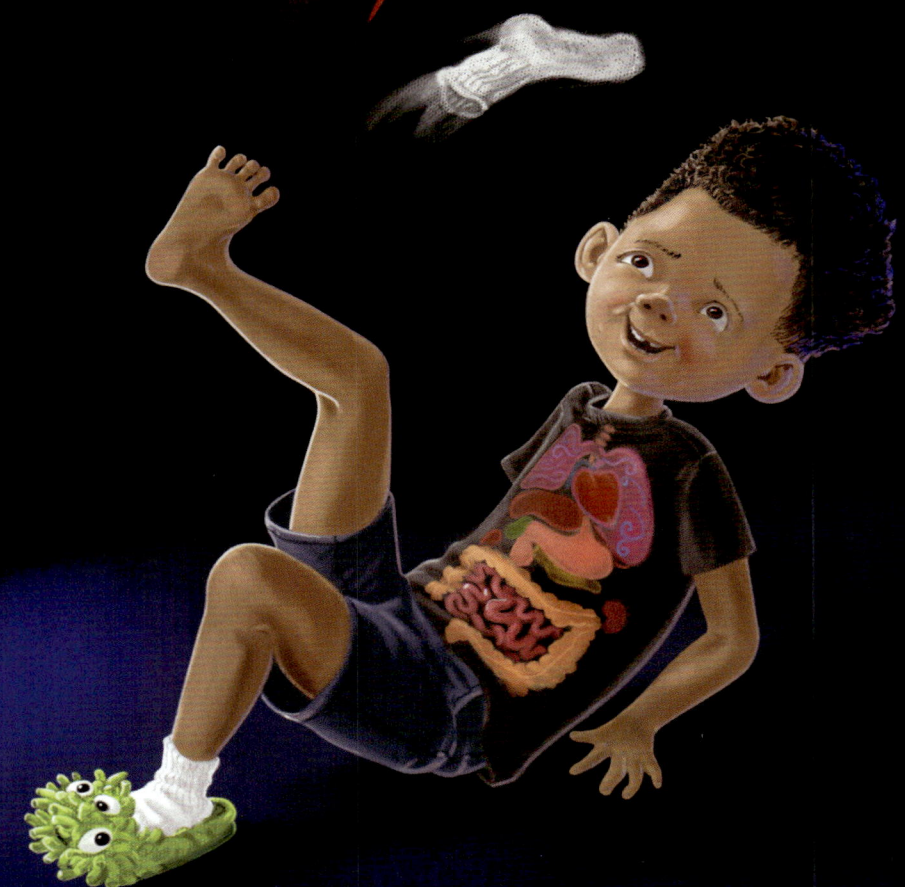

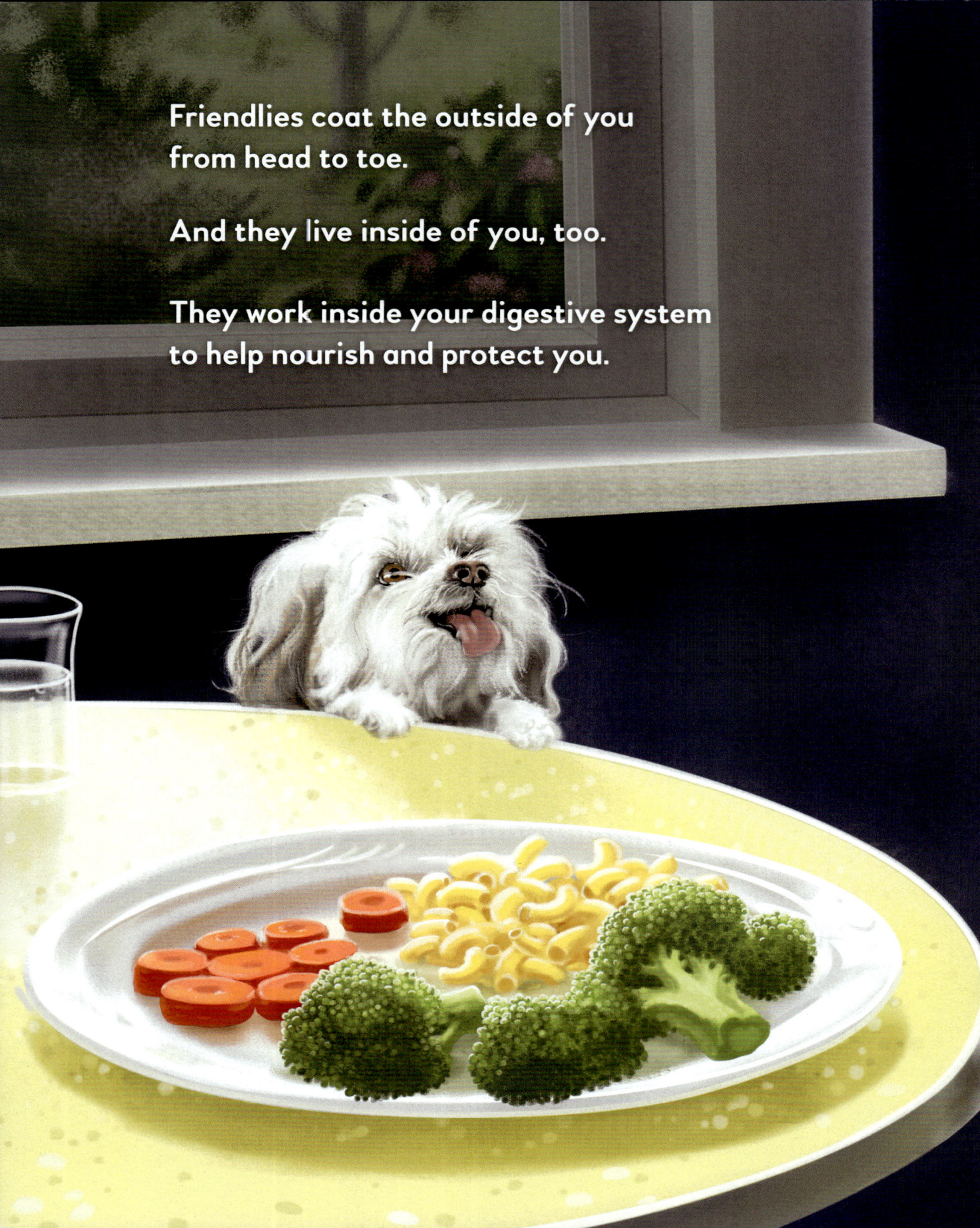

Friendlies coat the outside of you from head to toe.

And they live inside of you, too.

They work inside your digestive system to help nourish and protect you.

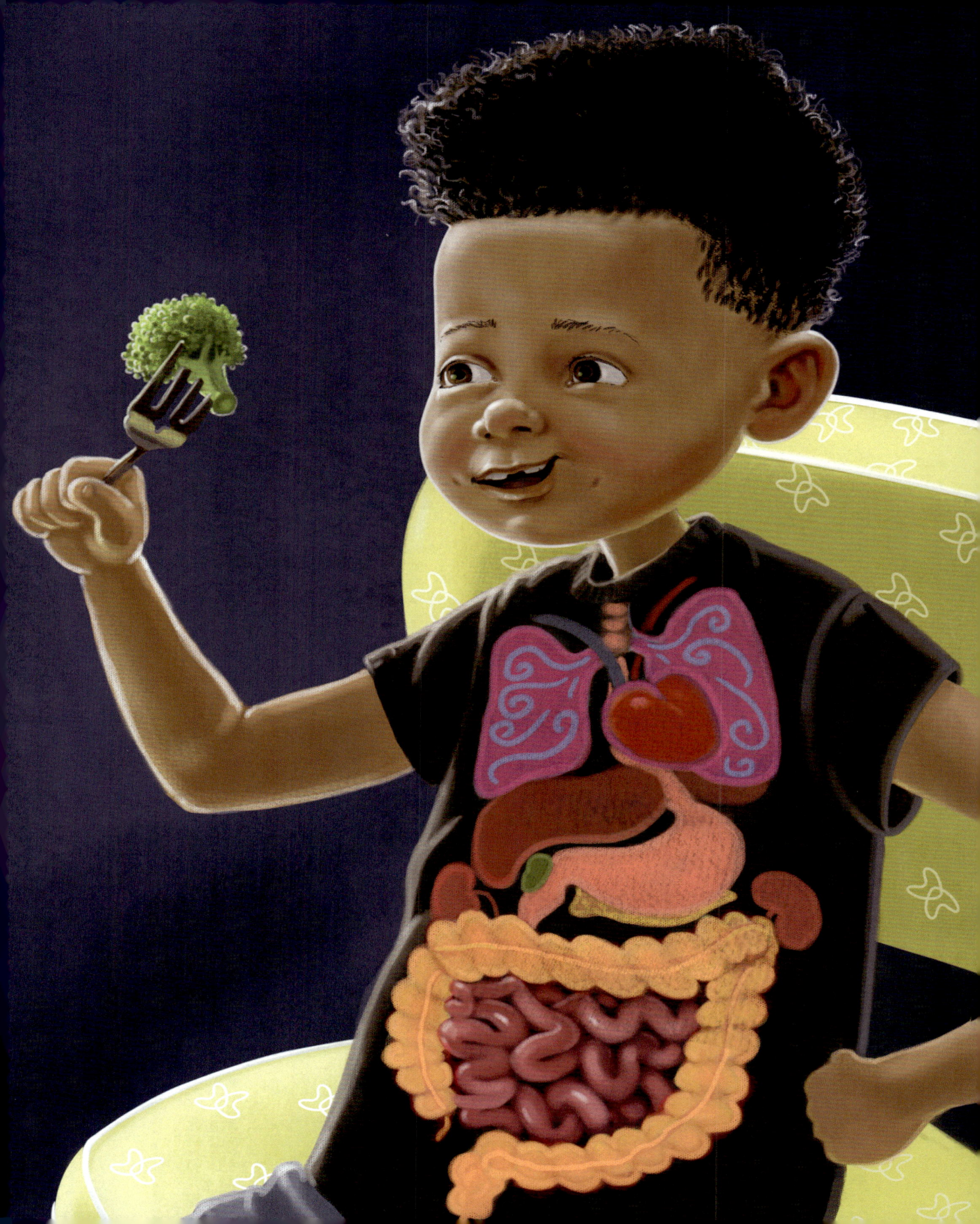

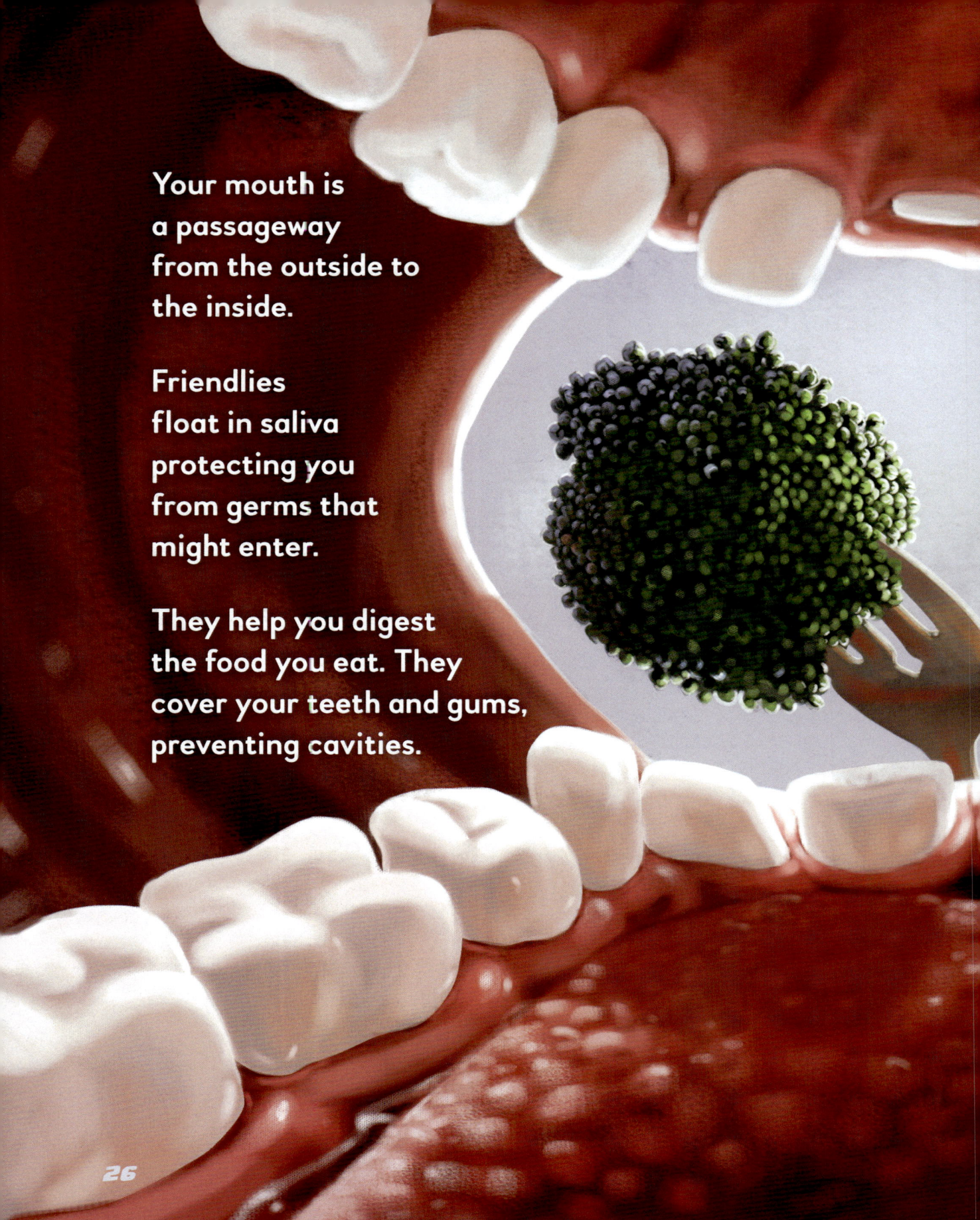

Your mouth is a passageway from the outside to the inside.

Friendlies float in saliva protecting you from germs that might enter.

They help you digest the food you eat. They cover your teeth and gums, preventing cavities.

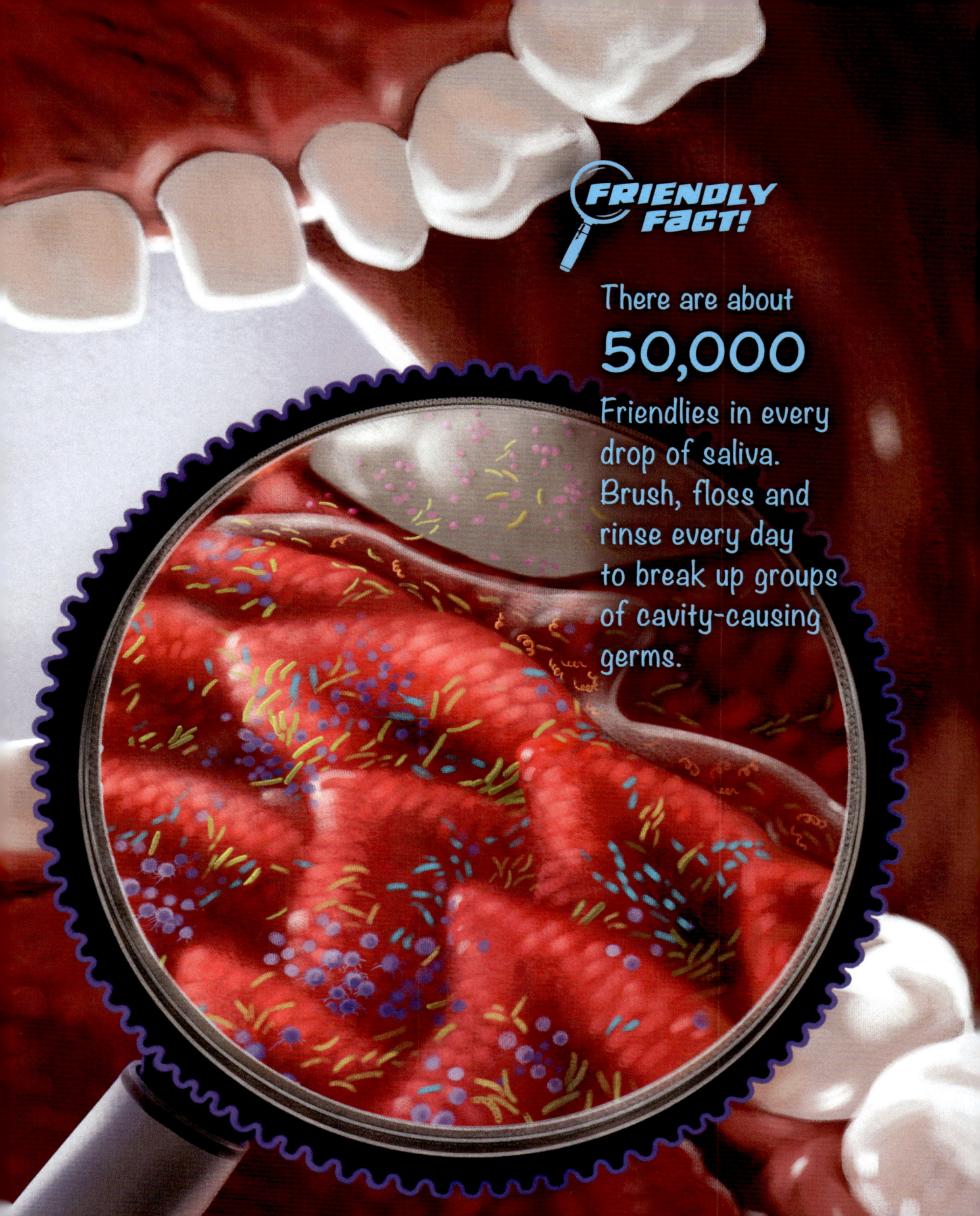

FRIENDLY FACT!

There are about **50,000** Friendlies in every drop of saliva. Brush, floss and rinse every day to break up groups of cavity-causing germs.

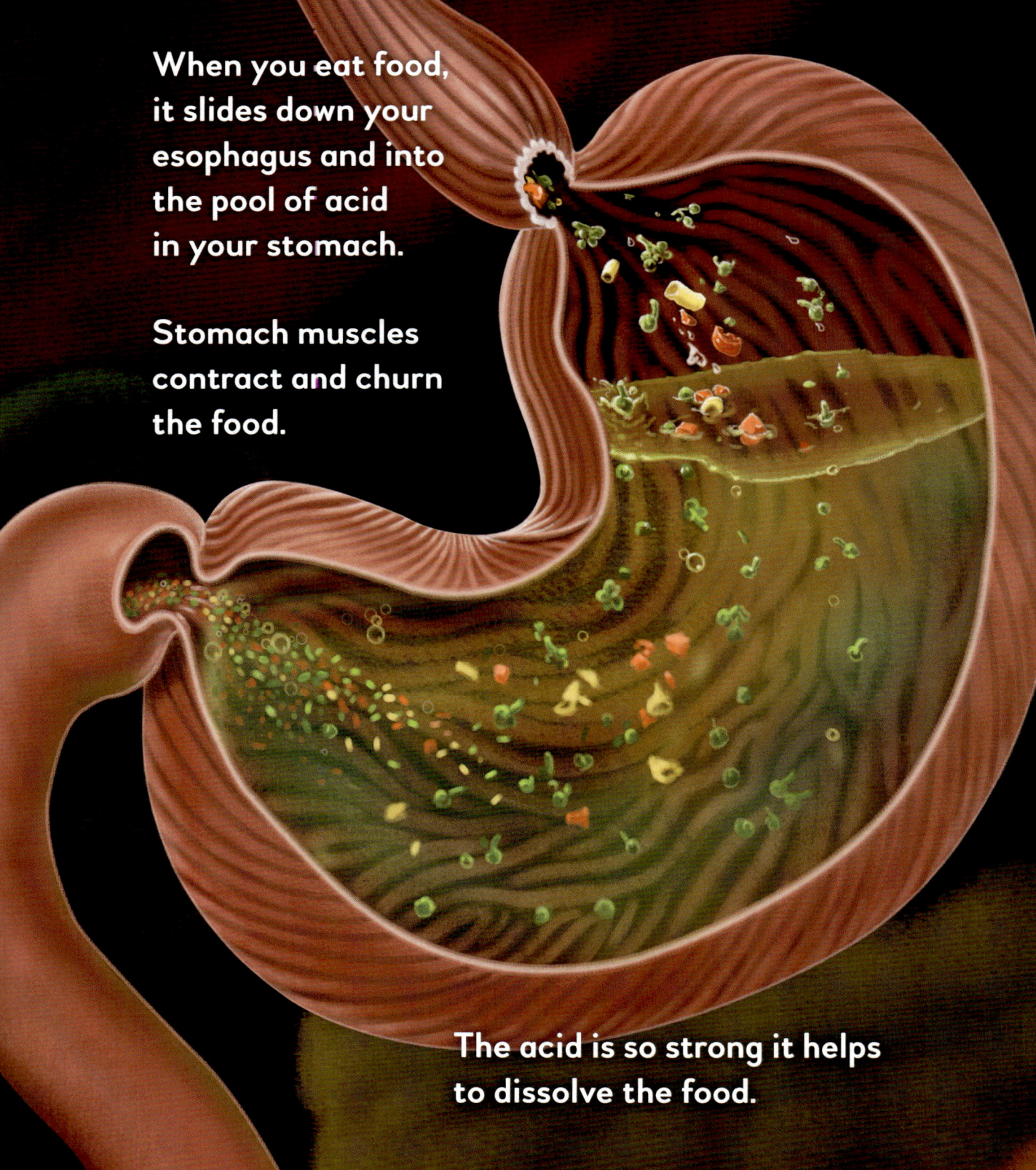

When you eat food, it slides down your esophagus and into the pool of acid in your stomach.

Stomach muscles contract and churn the food.

The acid is so strong it helps to dissolve the food.

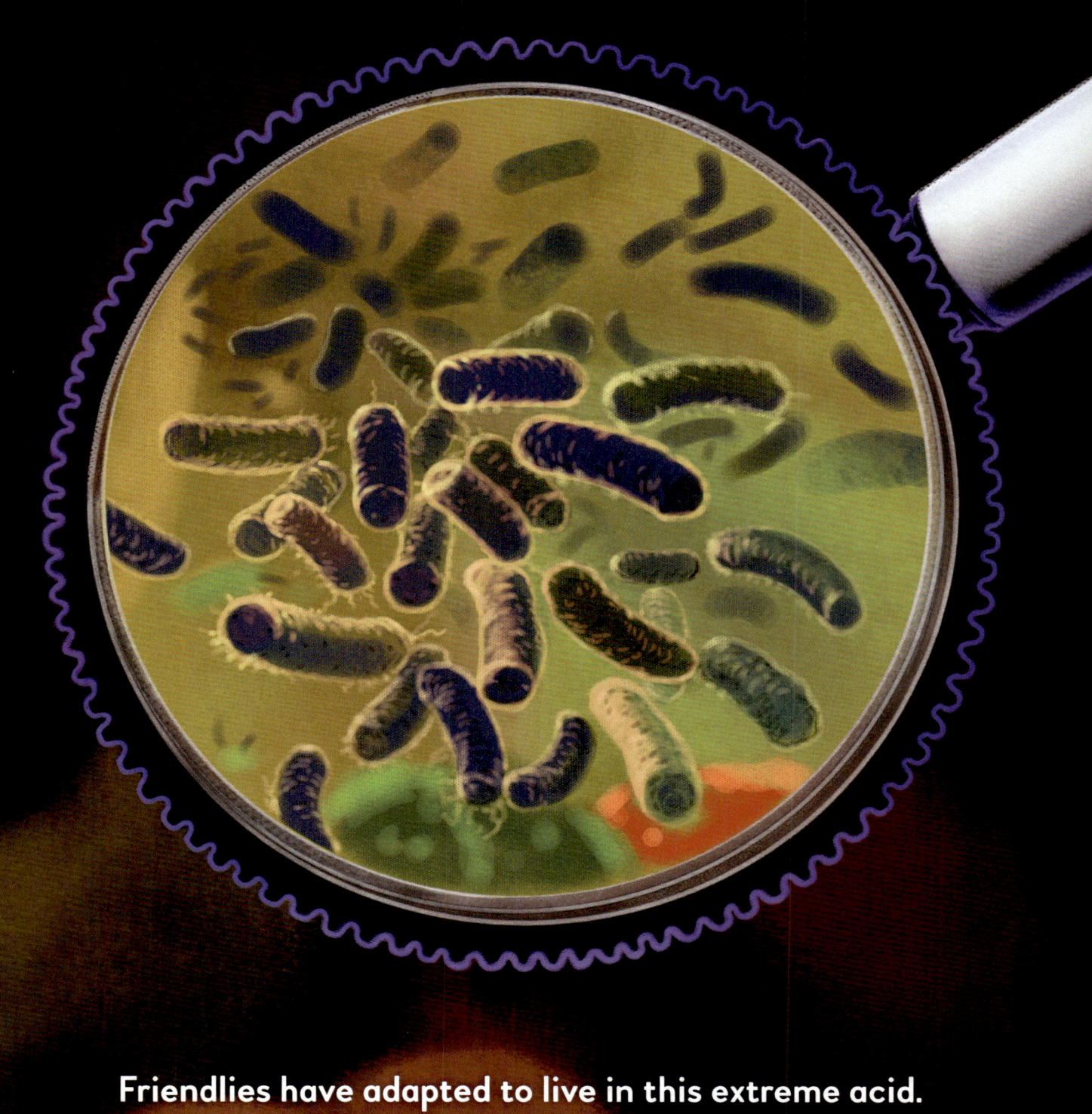

Friendlies have adapted to live in this extreme acid.
In fact, they are called "acid-loving" or acidophilus.

As the acid mush enters the small intestine, **enzymes** pour in from the **pancreas** and **gallbladder** to help digest the food.

They neutralize the strong acid creating the opposite **alkaline** habitat.

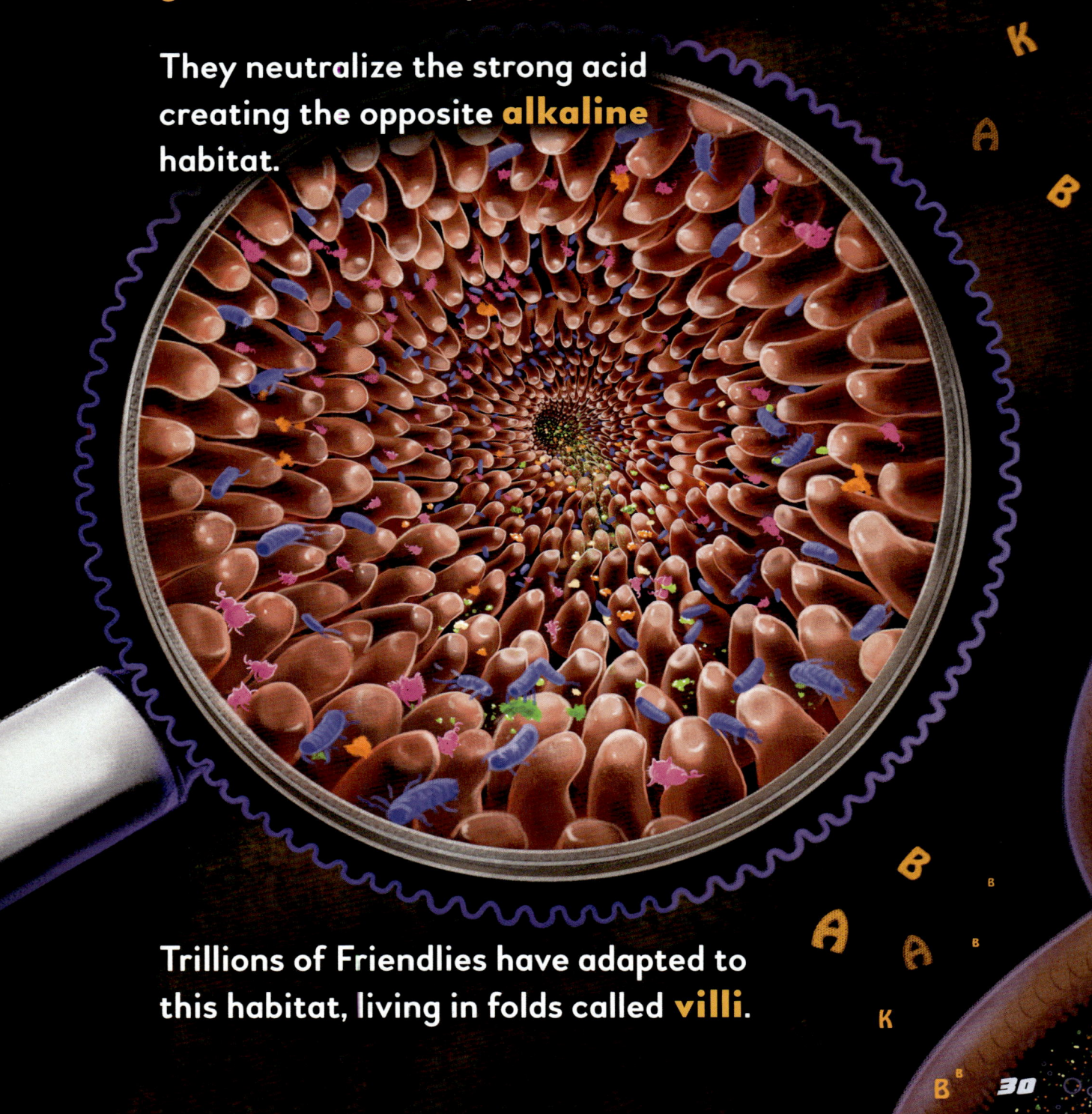

Trillions of Friendlies have adapted to this habitat, living in folds called **villi**.

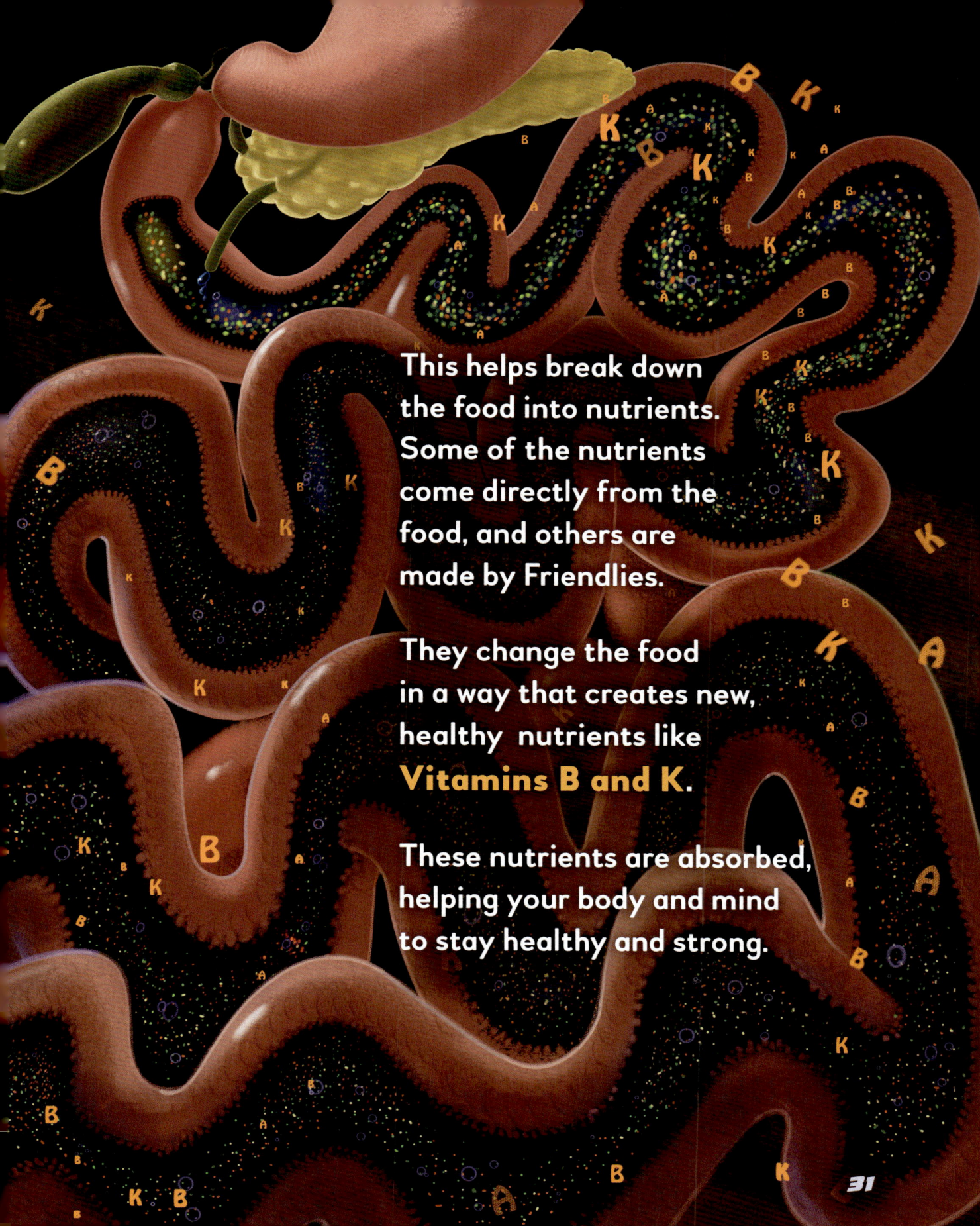

This helps break down the food into nutrients. Some of the nutrients come directly from the food, and others are made by Friendlies.

They change the food in a way that creates new, healthy nutrients like **Vitamins B and K.**

These nutrients are absorbed, helping your body and mind to stay healthy and strong.

Once most of the nutrients are absorbed, the mushy liquid moves to the colon. Water is absorbed back into the body and the waste becomes more solid.

Friendlies live on the inner lining of the colon, creating a protective film that makes it hard for germs to hang on.

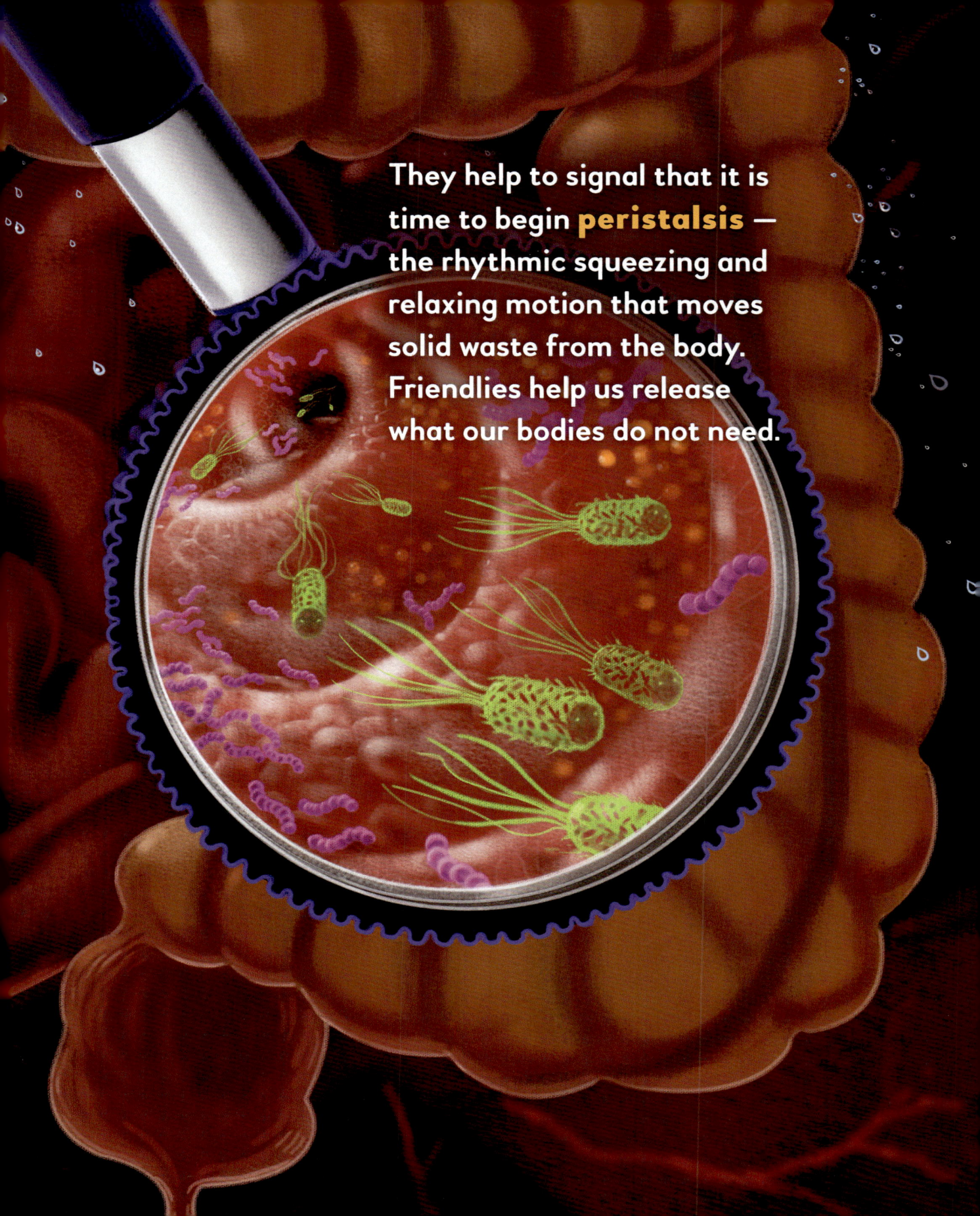

They help to signal that it is time to begin **peristalsis** — the rhythmic squeezing and relaxing motion that moves solid waste from the body. Friendlies help us release what our bodies do not need.

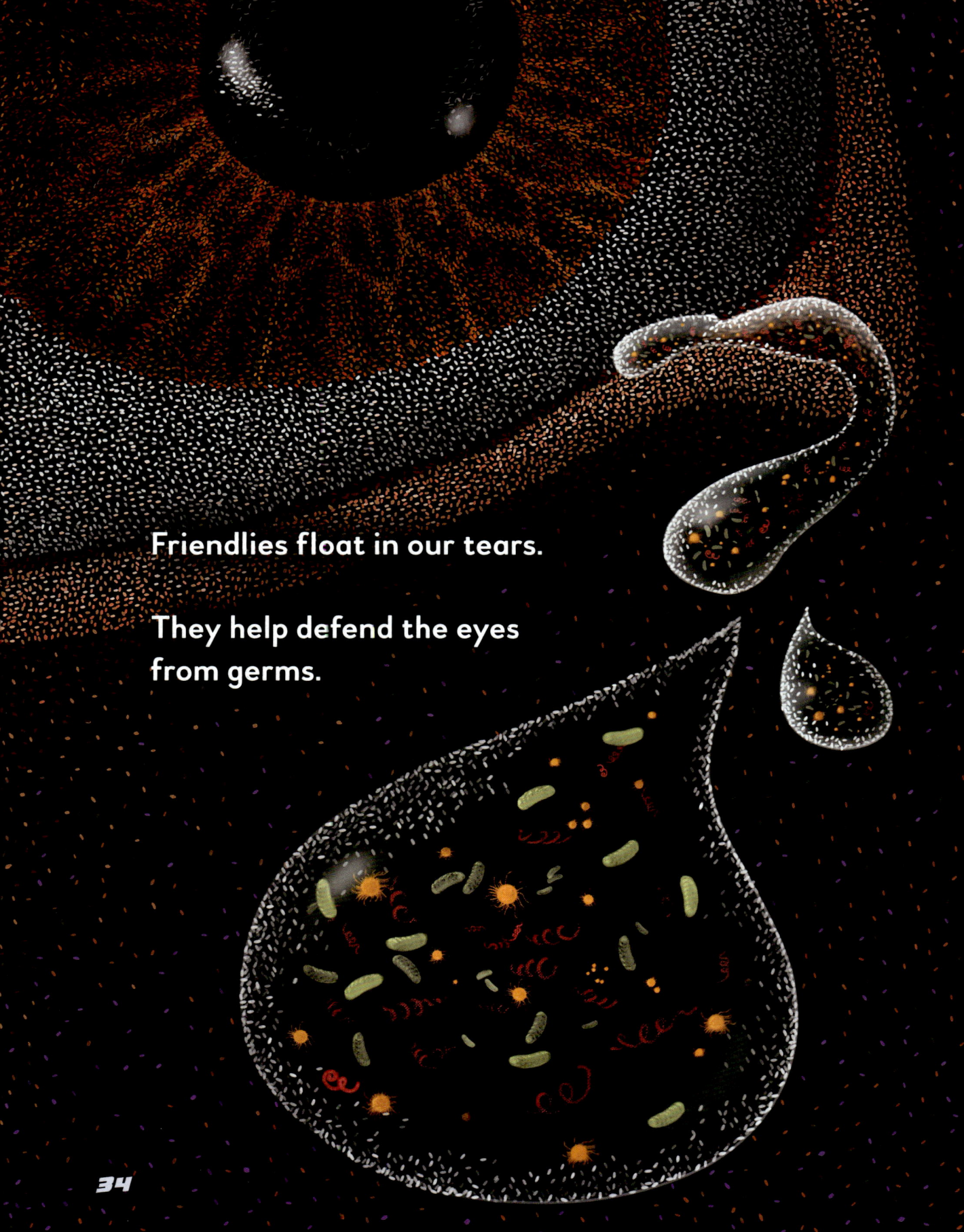

Friendlies float in our tears.

They help defend the eyes from germs.

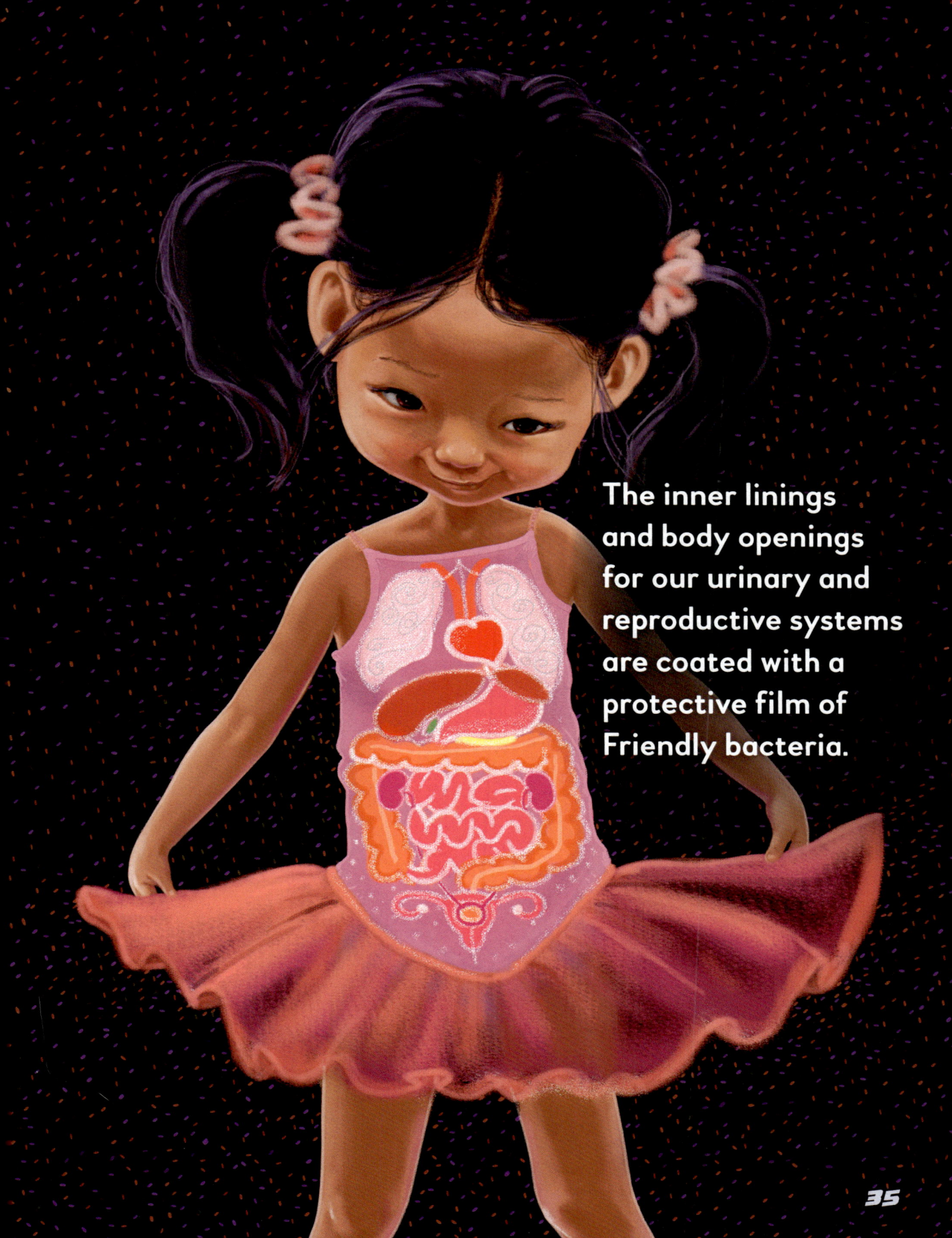

The inner linings and body openings for our urinary and reproductive systems are coated with a protective film of Friendly bacteria.

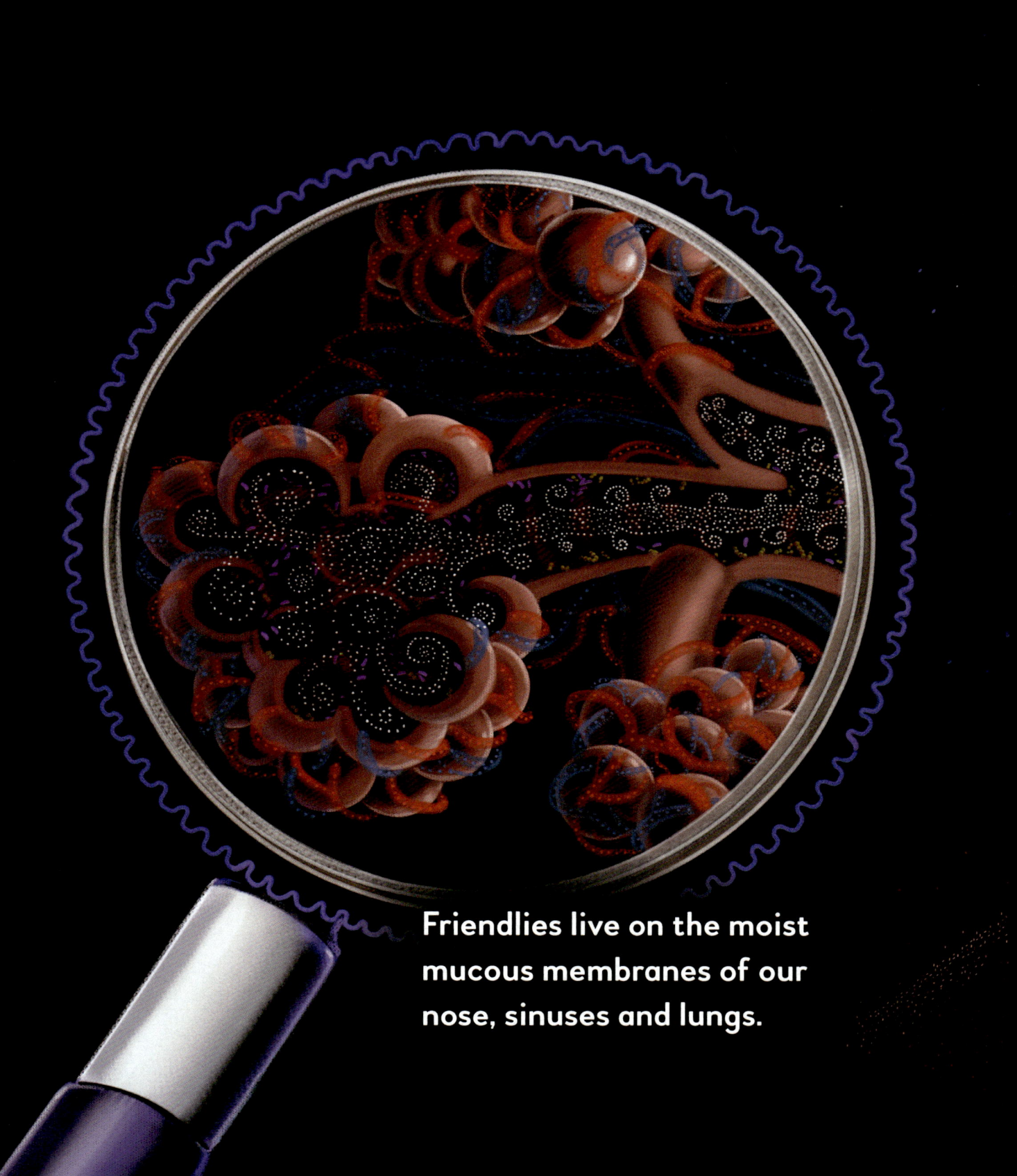

Friendlies live on the moist mucous membranes of our nose, sinuses and lungs.

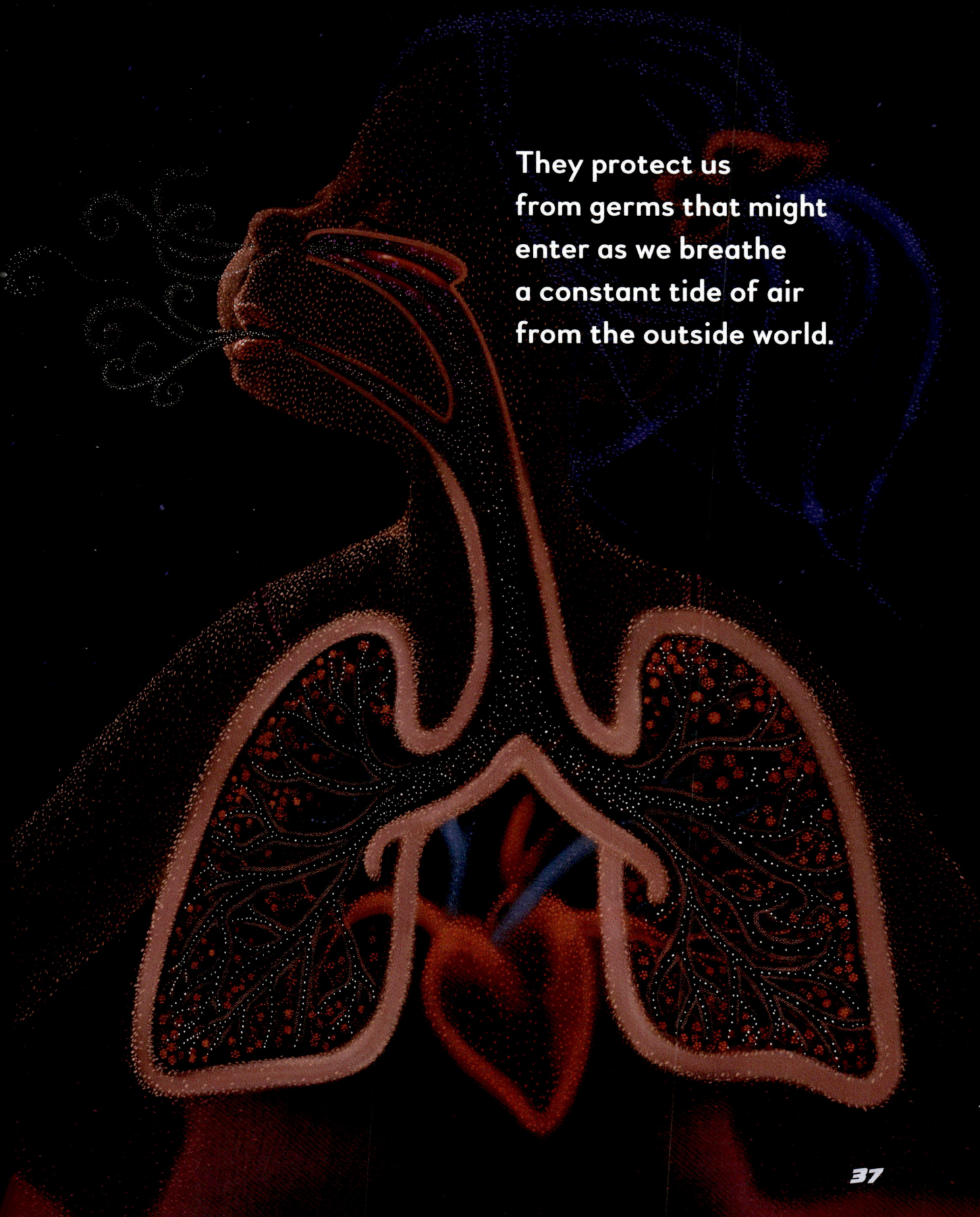
They protect us from germs that might enter as we breathe a constant tide of air from the outside world.

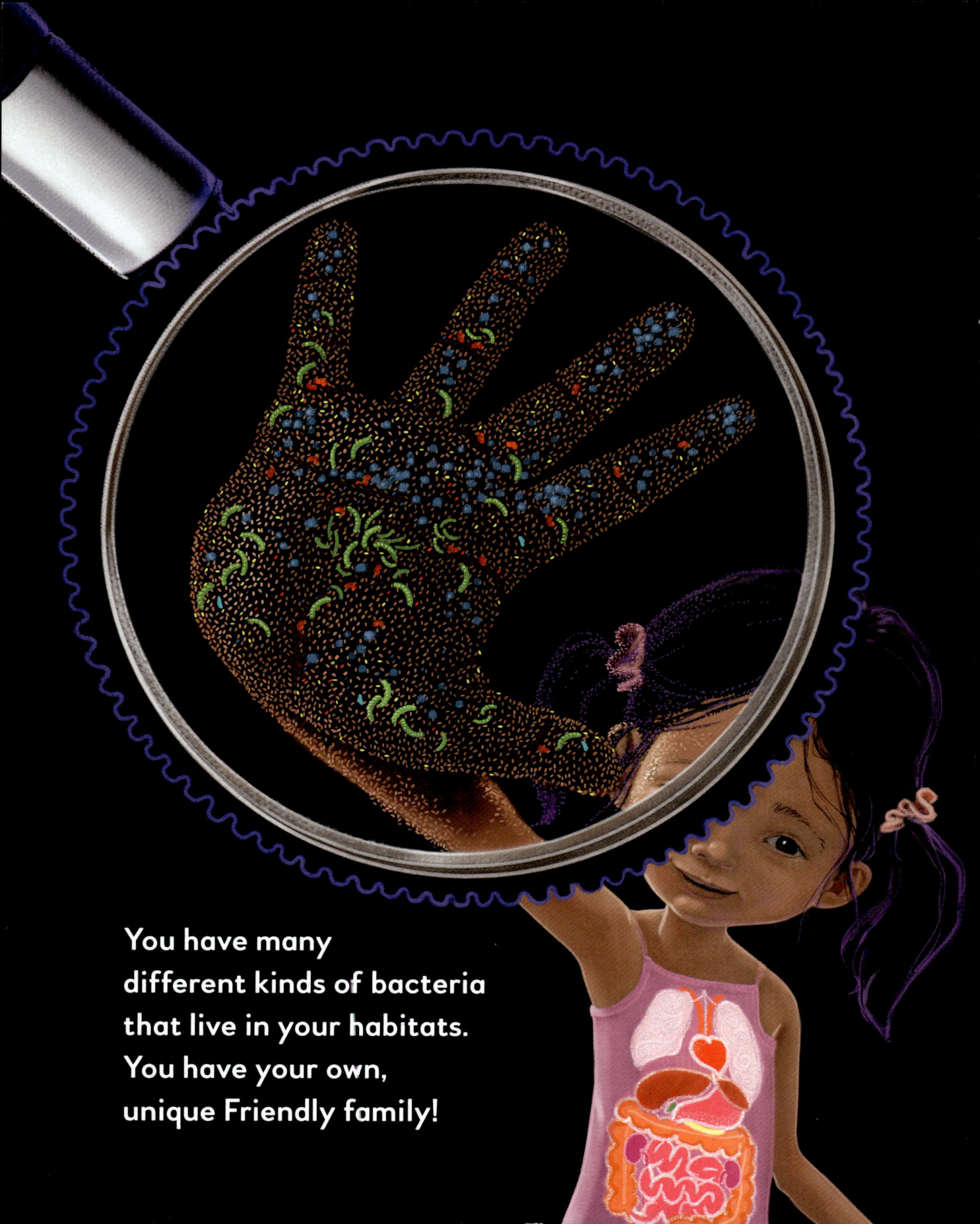

You have many different kinds of bacteria that live in your habitats. You have your own, unique Friendly family!

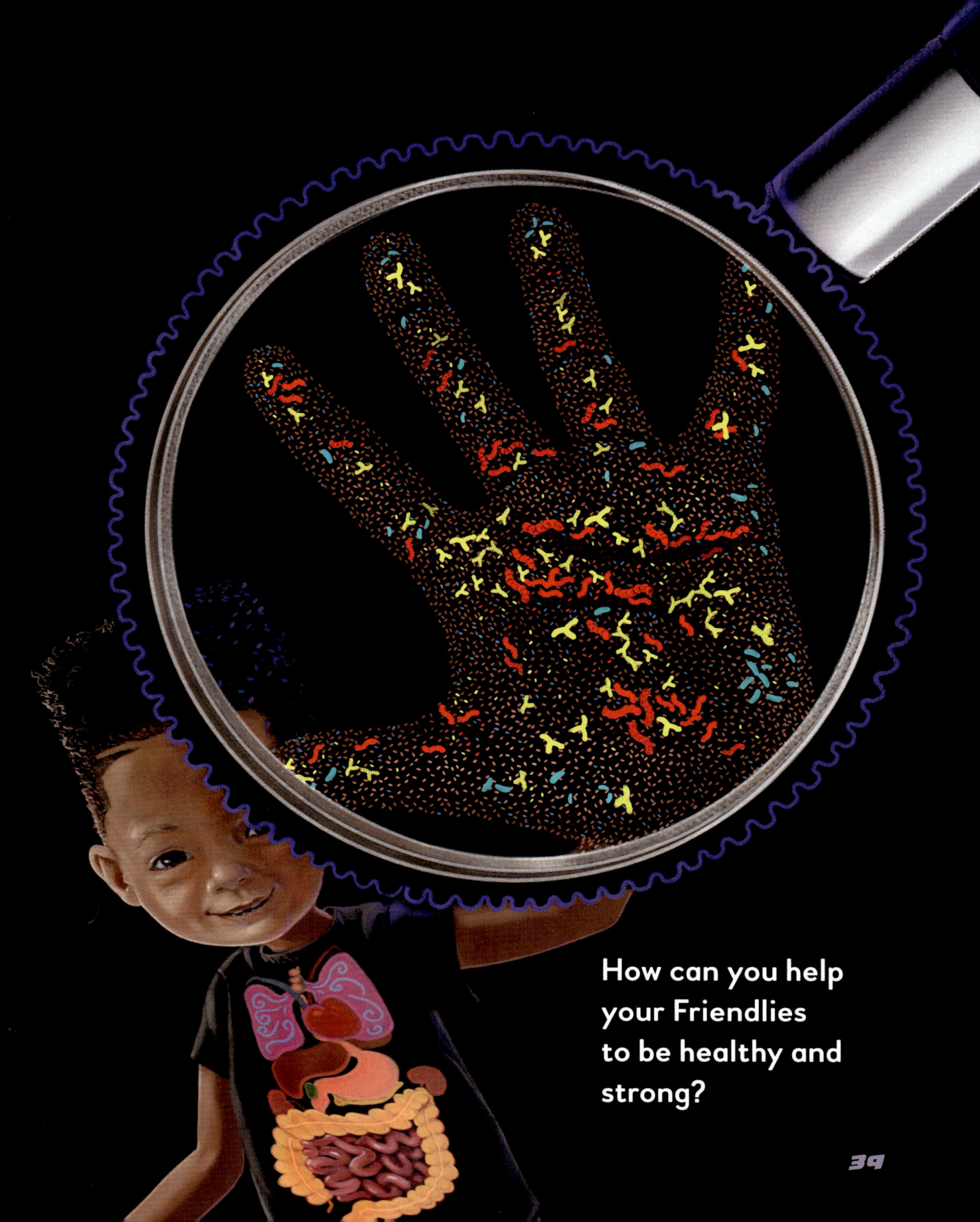

How can you help your Friendlies to be healthy and strong?

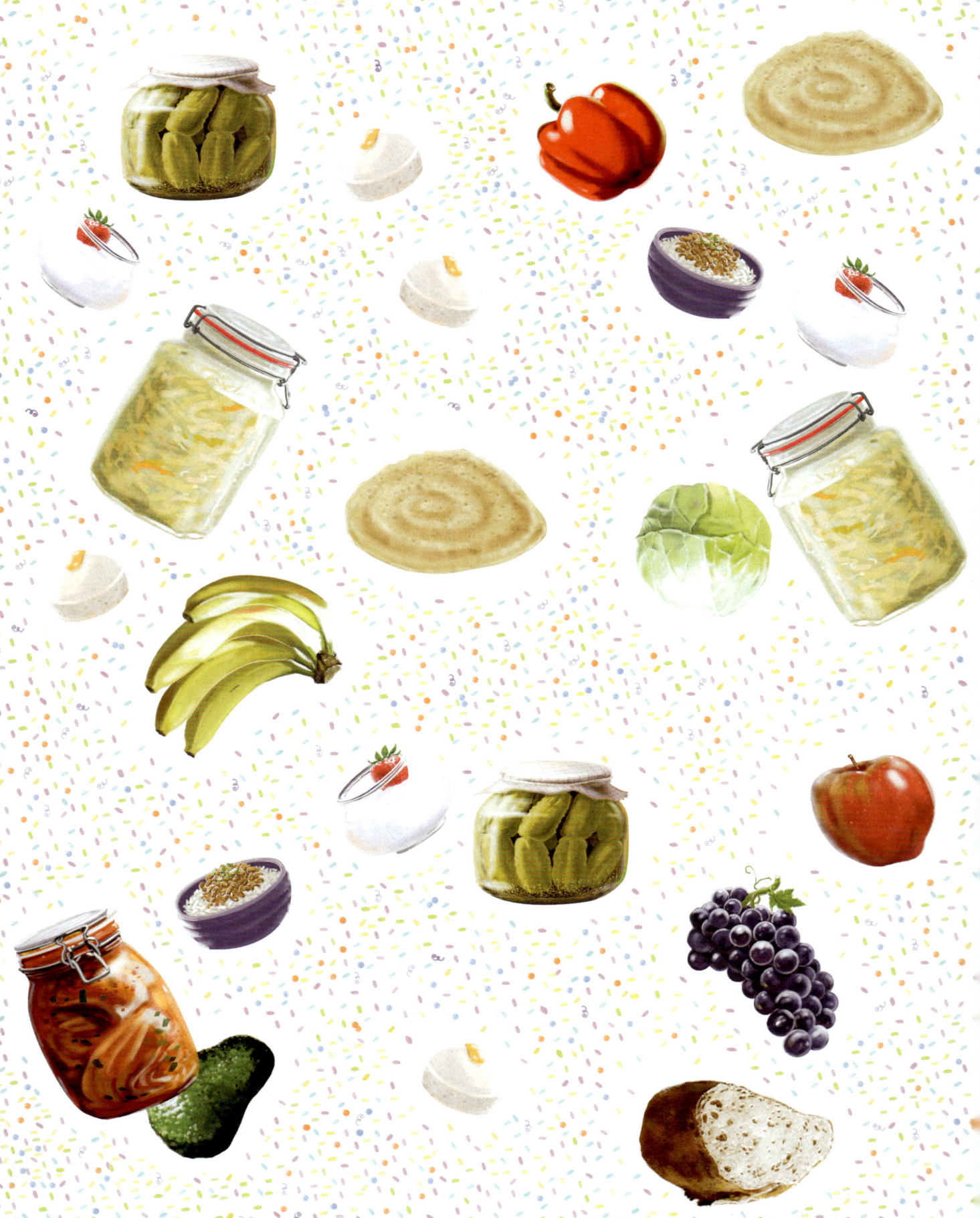

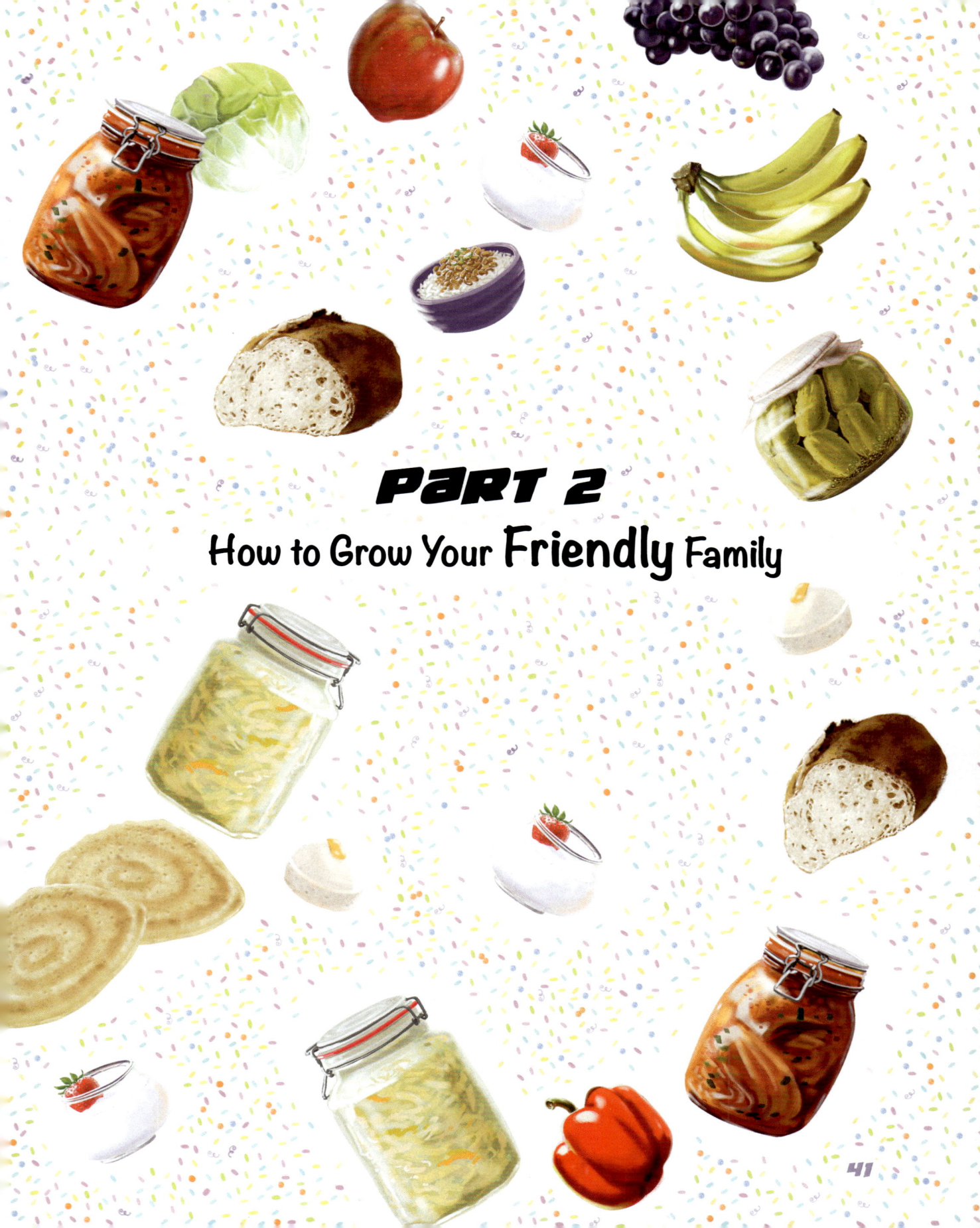

PART 2
How to Grow Your Friendly Family

You can grow your Friendly Family with

Fiber and
Cultured foods.

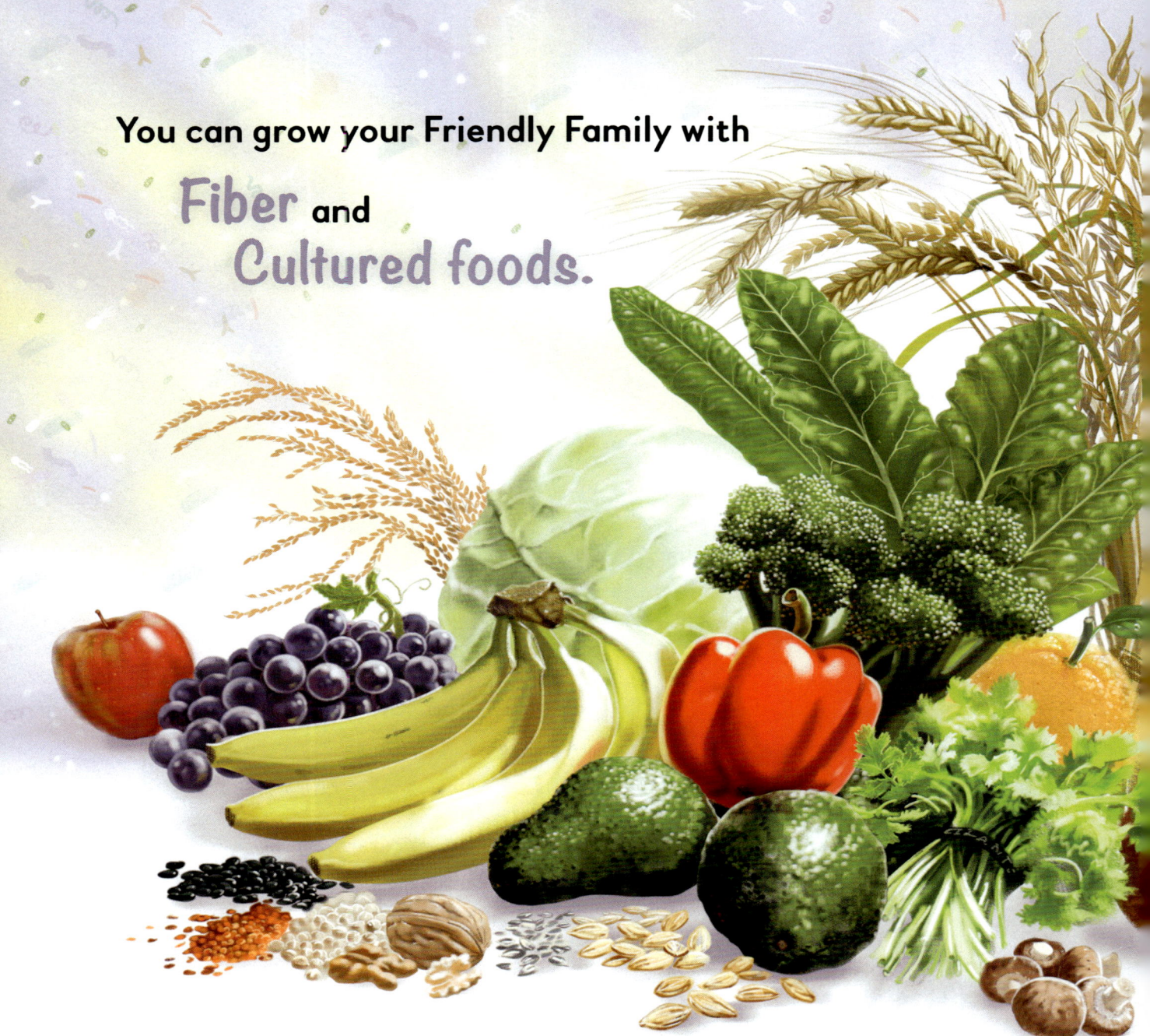

What is Fiber?

Plant foods like vegetables, fruits, nuts and seeds, beans and grains all have fiber, a kind of plant starch. These foods are called pre-biotics, because they provide energy to Friendlies to keep them strong.

What are Cultured foods?

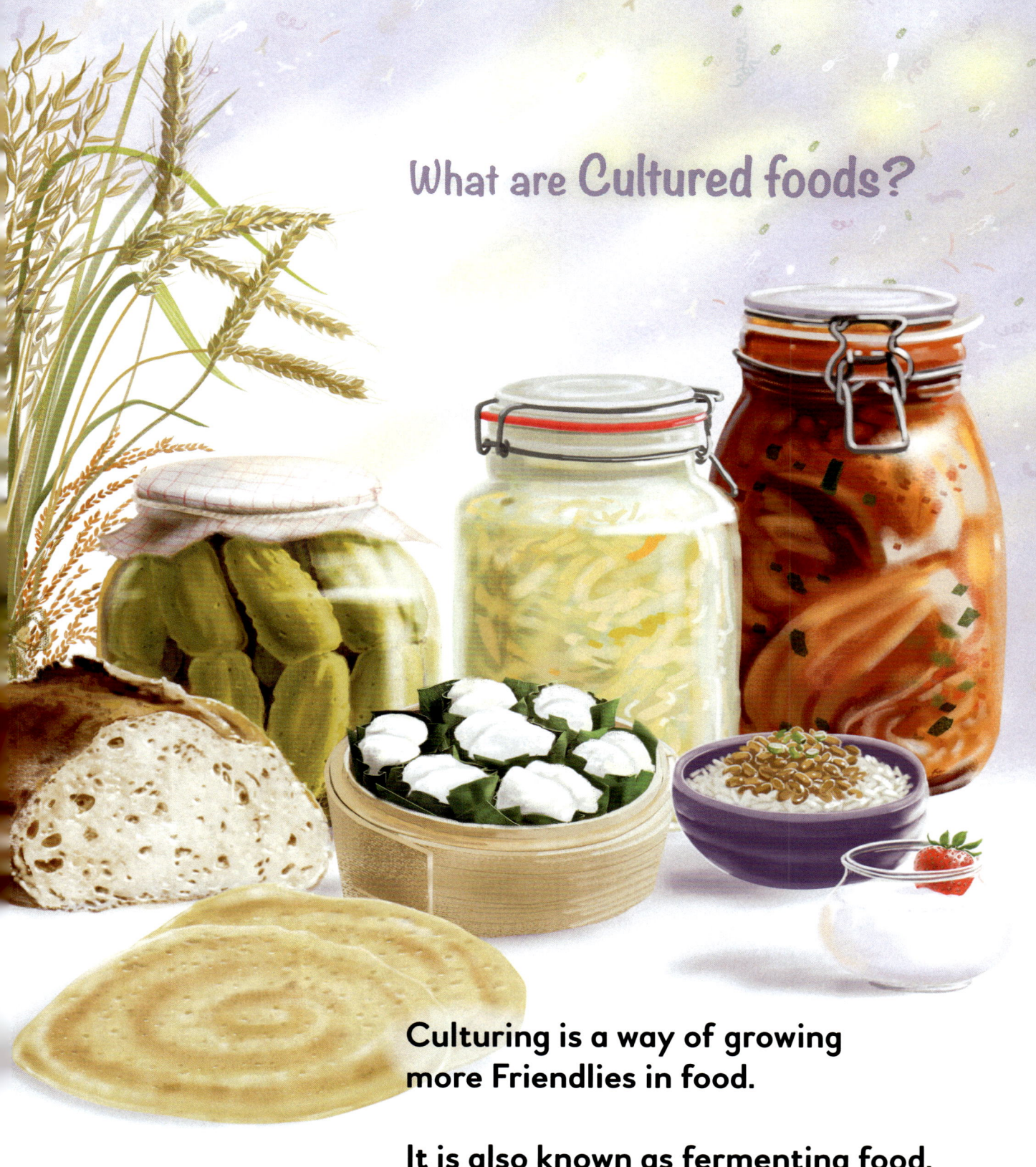

Culturing is a way of growing more Friendlies in food.

It is also known as fermenting food.

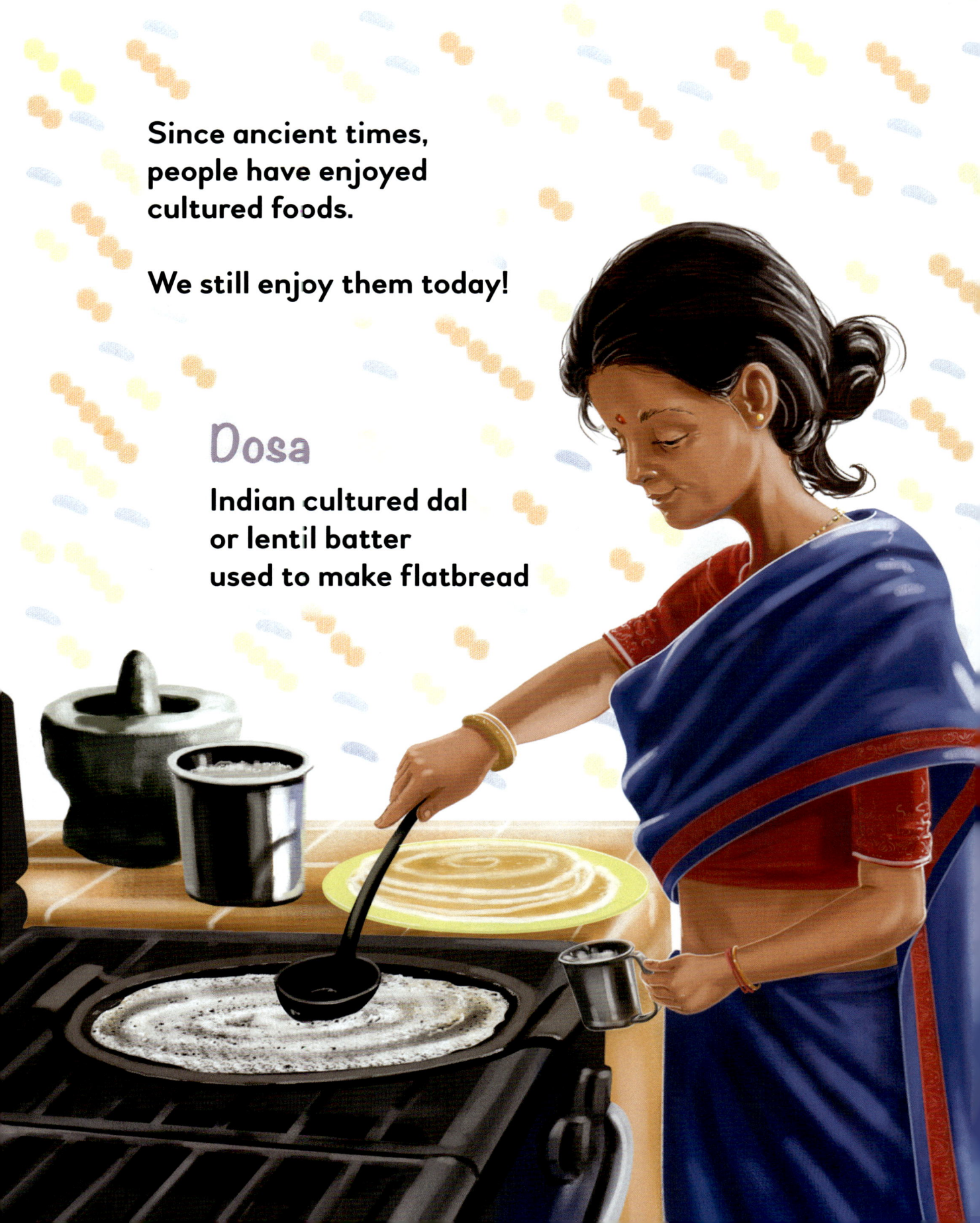

Since ancient times, people have enjoyed cultured foods.

We still enjoy them today!

Dosa

Indian cultured dal or lentil batter used to make flatbread

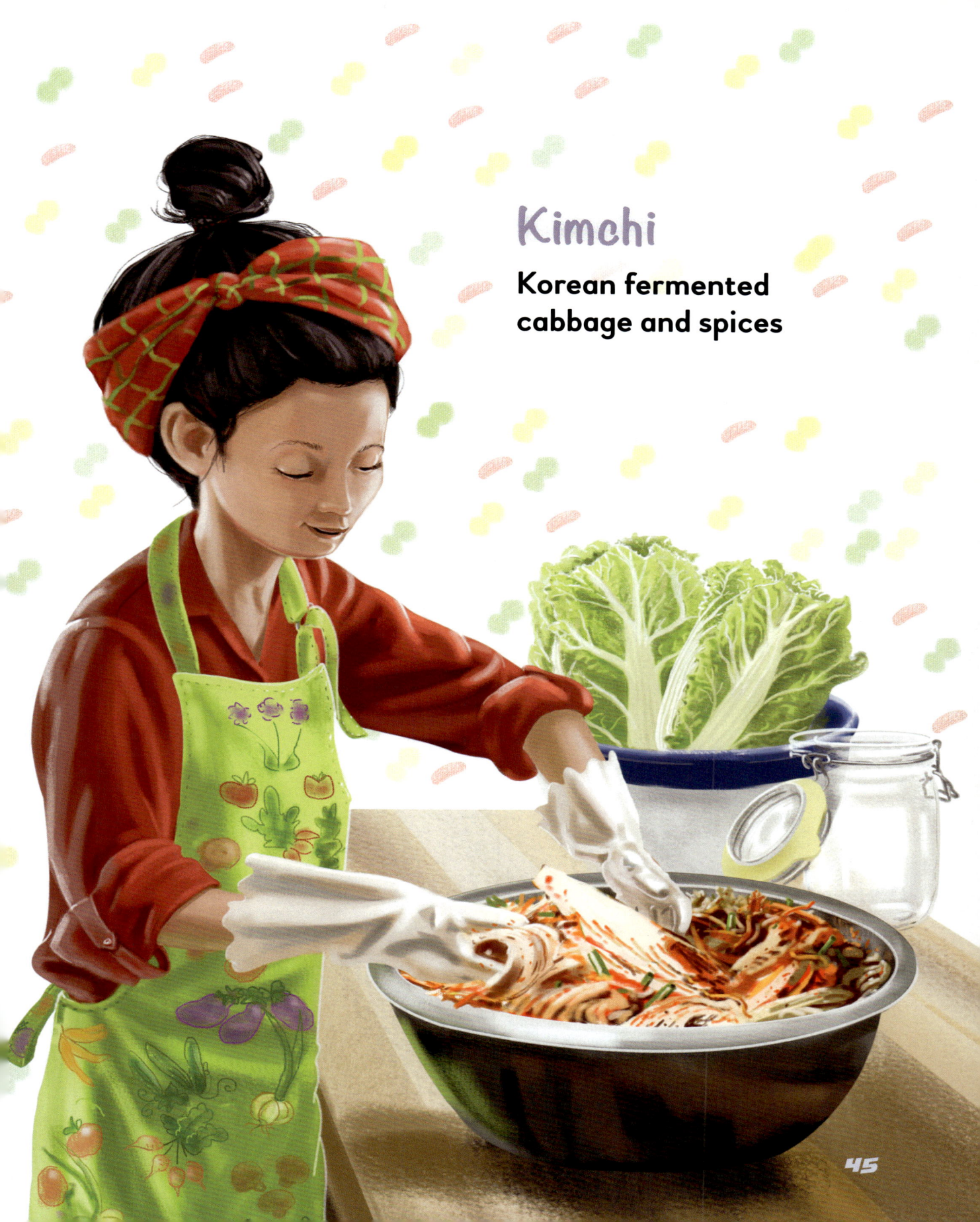

Kimchi

Korean fermented cabbage and spices

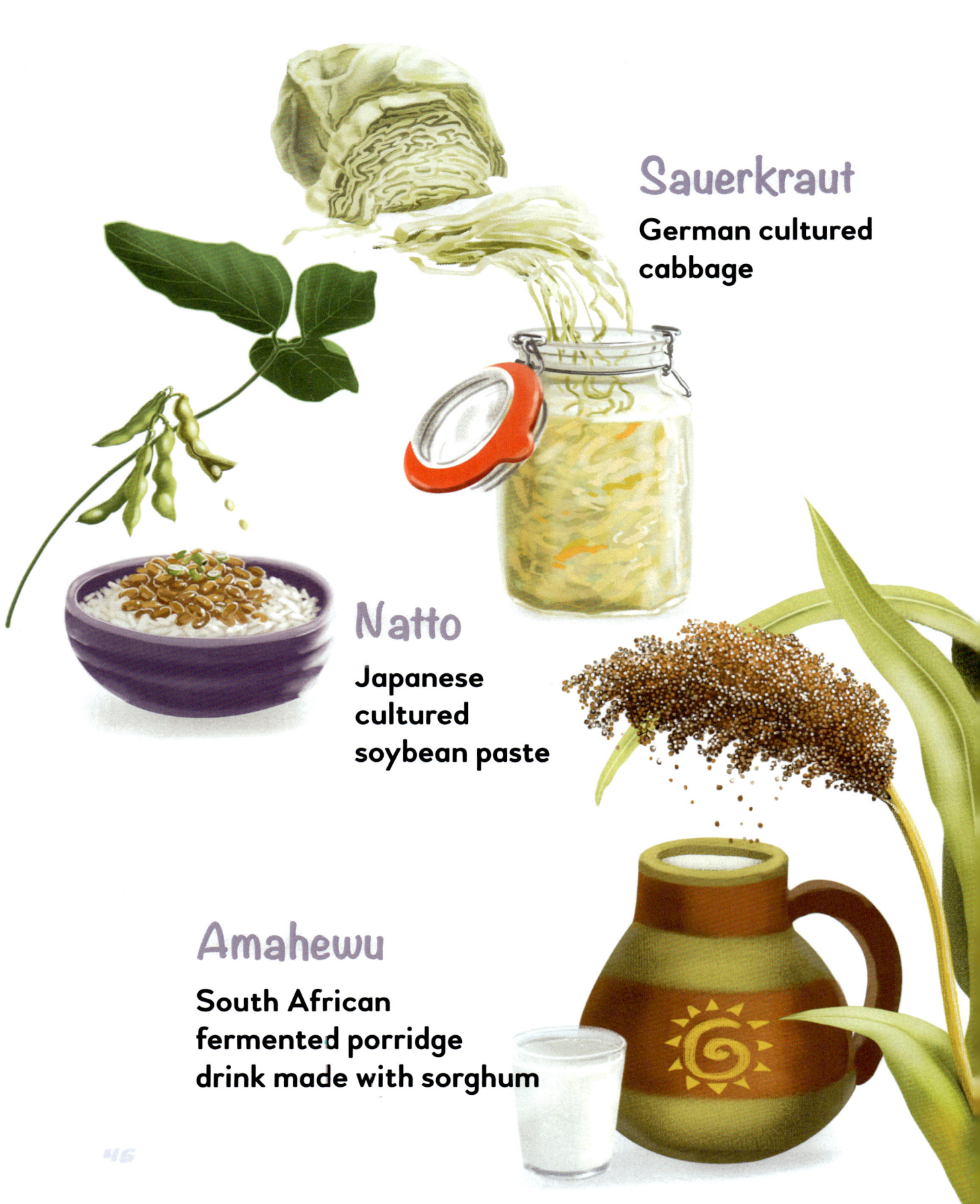

Sauerkraut
German cultured cabbage

Natto
Japanese cultured soybean paste

Amahewu
South African fermented porridge drink made with sorghum

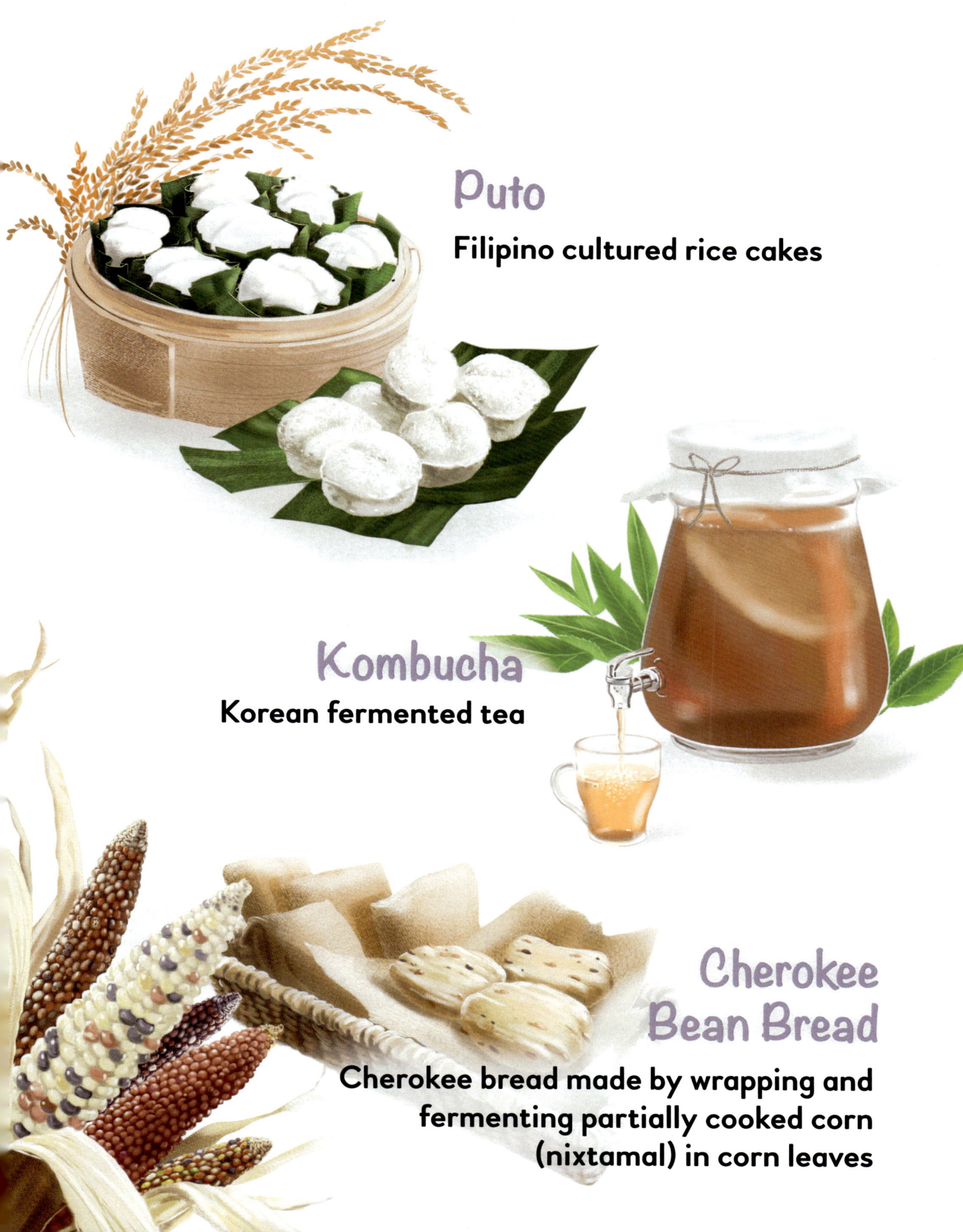

Puto
Filipino cultured rice cakes

Kombucha
Korean fermented tea

Cherokee Bean Bread
Cherokee bread made by wrapping and fermenting partially cooked corn (nixtamal) in corn leaves

How do we culture food?

There are 4 main steps!

1. **Add Friendlies (also known as a "starter culture")**

   You can add a spoonful of cultured food, (such as yogurt) or let Friendlies settle onto the food from the air (sometimes called "wild cultures.")

2. **Feed them.**

   Check that there is sugar to feed the Friendlies. (They will digest all the sugar and there will not be any left in the cultured food.)

3. Cover them.

Friendlies grow best in a warm, dark place.

4. Allow enough time.

Many cultured foods can be made overnight. Some take days, weeks or even years!

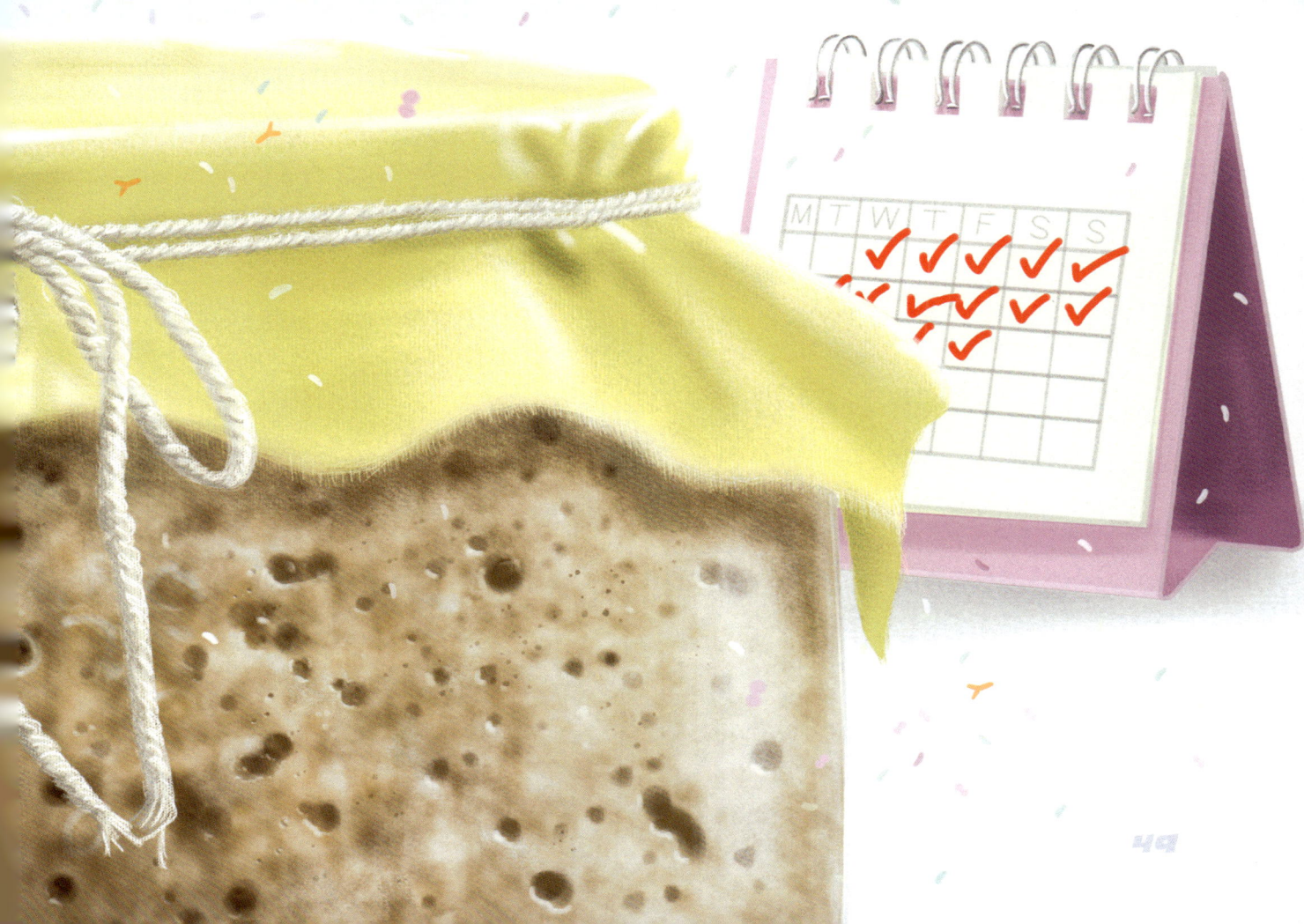

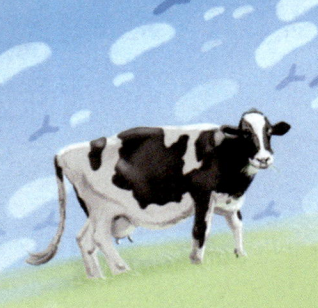

Yogurt

Try this recipe with a grown-up helper to make your own cultured food for you and your Friendlies.

Ingredients:

2 cups milk
(organic dairy or non-dairy milk)

A culture
3 Tbs. yogurt already made or packaged starter culture (dairy or non-dairy)

Sweetener (Optional)
Such as stevia, raw honey or agave nectar — to be added after the yogurt has cooled.

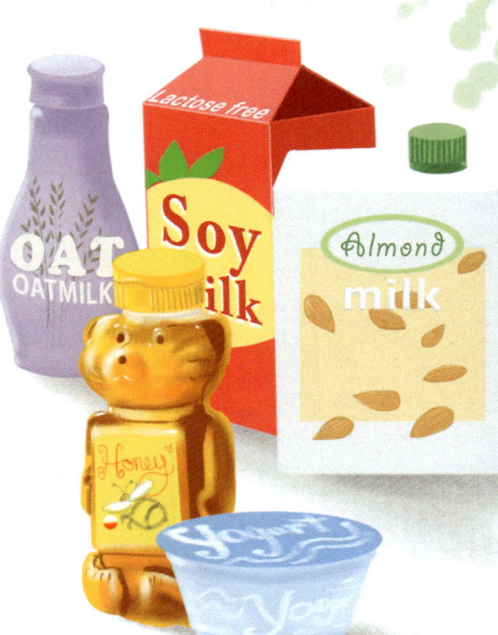

Supplies:

Clean containers to hold the milk — each should hold 1/2 cup (4 ounces).
(For example: 4 small glasses, jars, cups or bowls)

Clean cloth and rubber bands to cover the containers.

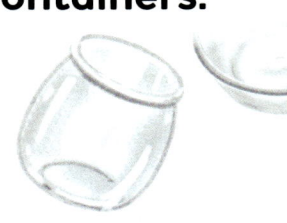
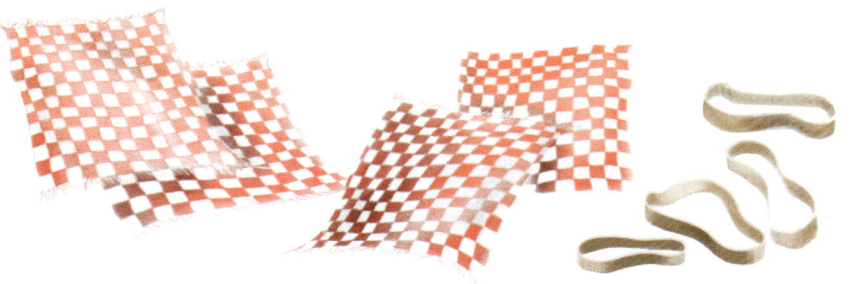

Steps:

1. Heat the milk, using a thermometer to 110º F or until it feels very warm to the touch

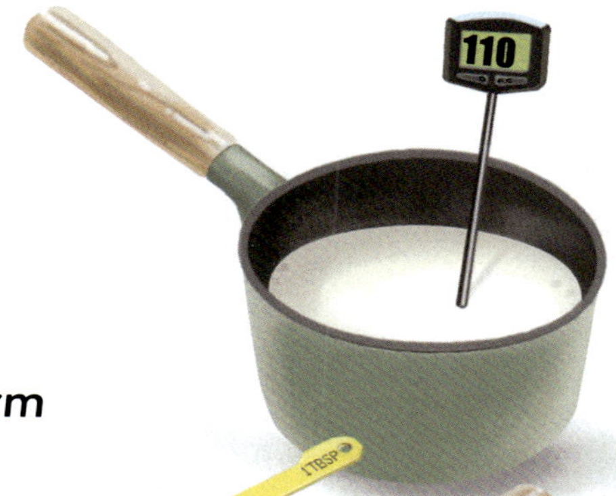

2. Stir the culture into the milk and mix well

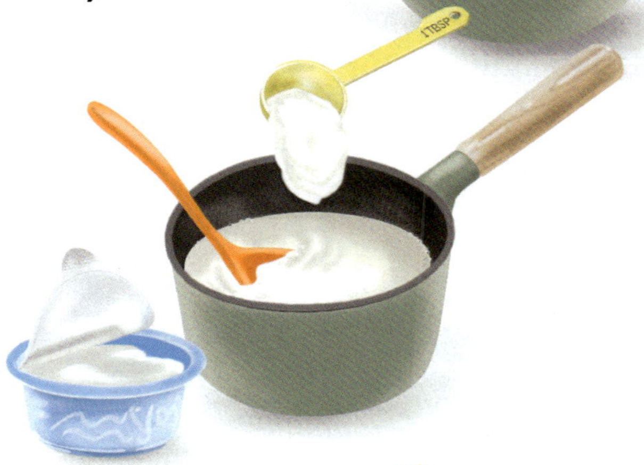

3. Pour the mixture into containers

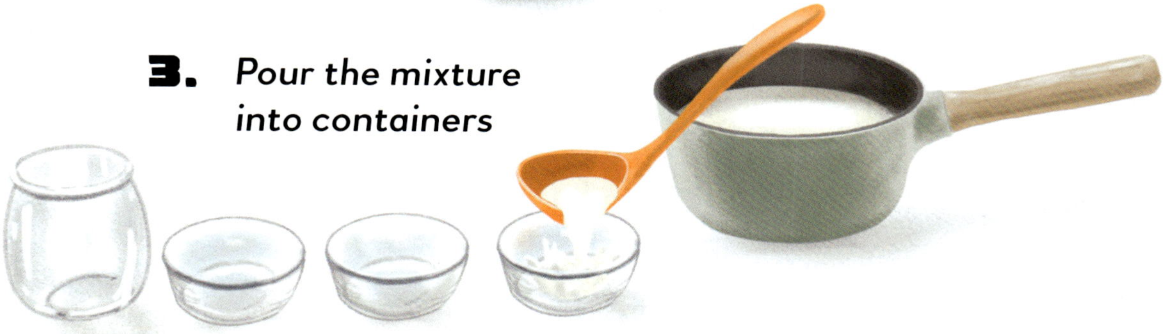

4. Cover the jar with a cloth or paper towel or loose lid (do not use a tight lid or the trapped air could cause the lid to pop off and the yogurt to spill out)

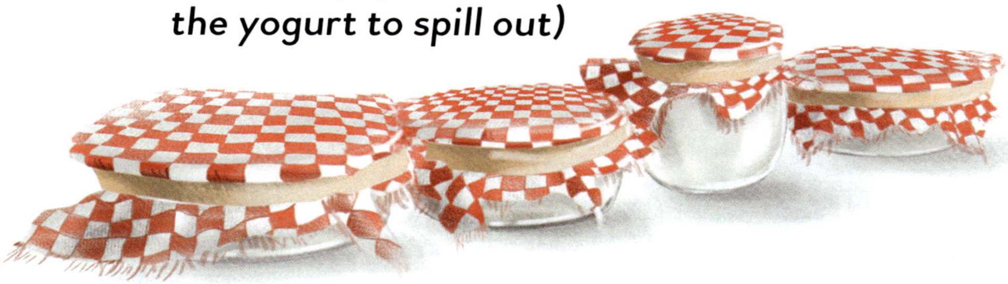

5. Keep in a warm place (about 110-115º F) for 5 to 10 hours (or overnight)

The yogurt is ready when it has thickened.

It should have a pleasant, lightly sour smell and taste.

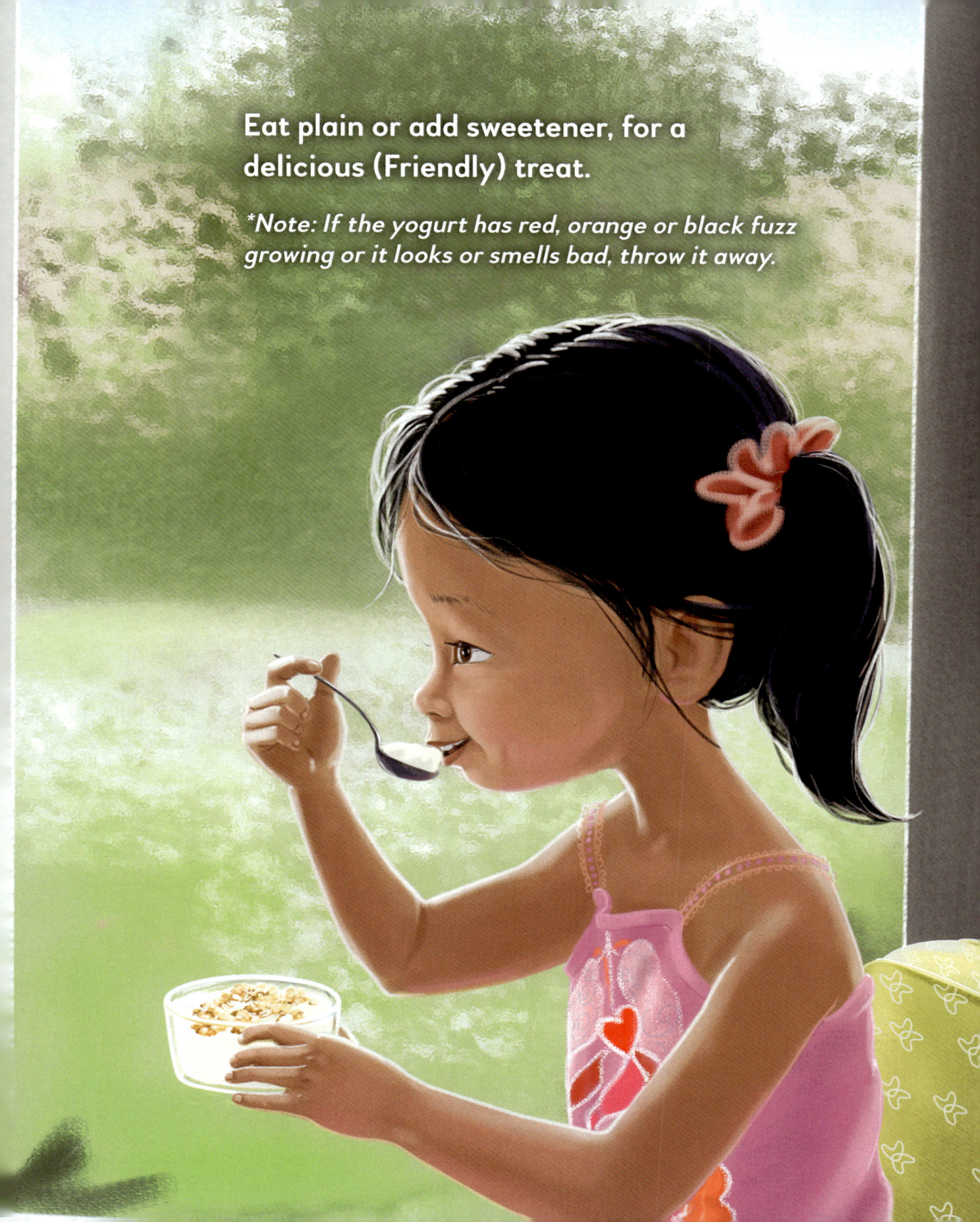

Now that you know about your Friendlies, what will you do?

☑ **Care for my body and mind**

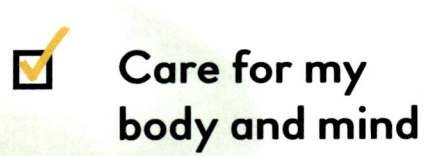

☑ **Brush *and* floss, making sure my teeth are clean before bed**

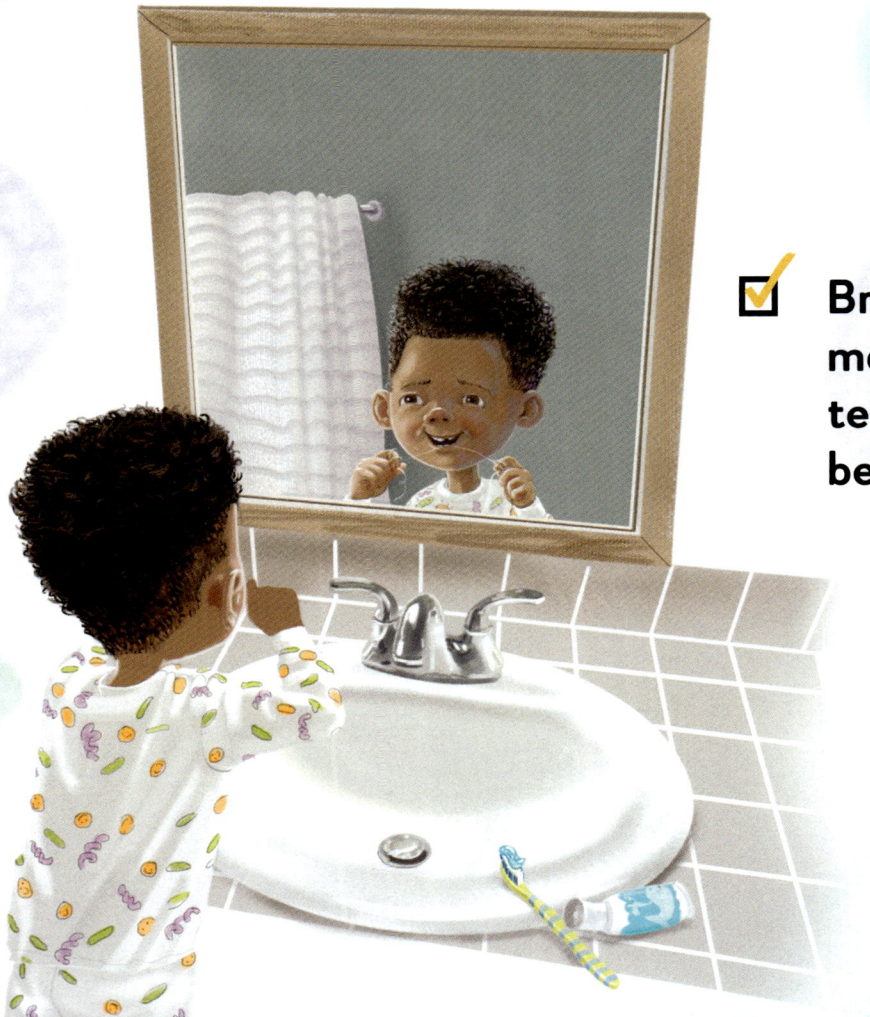

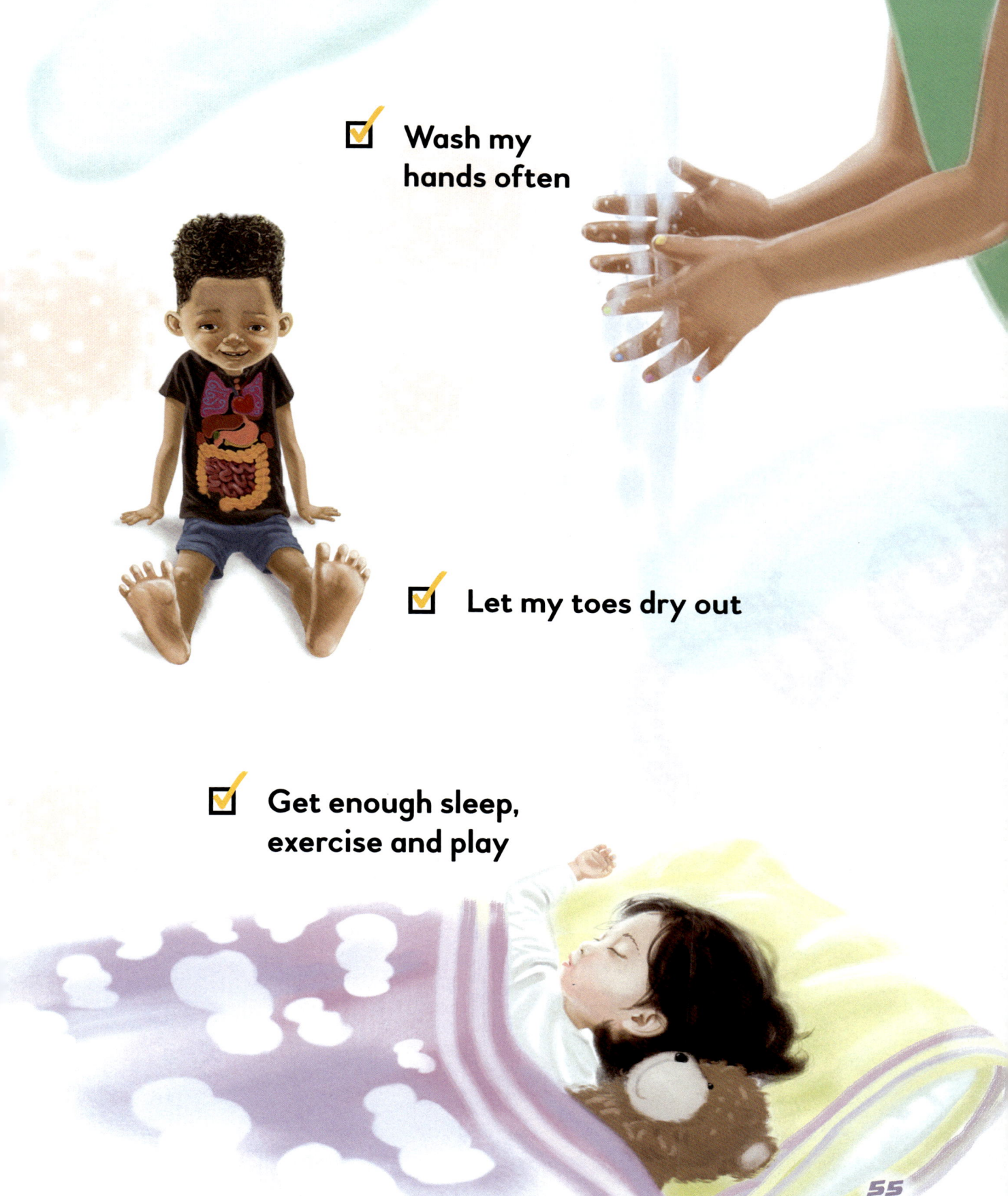

☑ Wash my hands often

☑ Let my toes dry out

☑ Get enough sleep, exercise and play

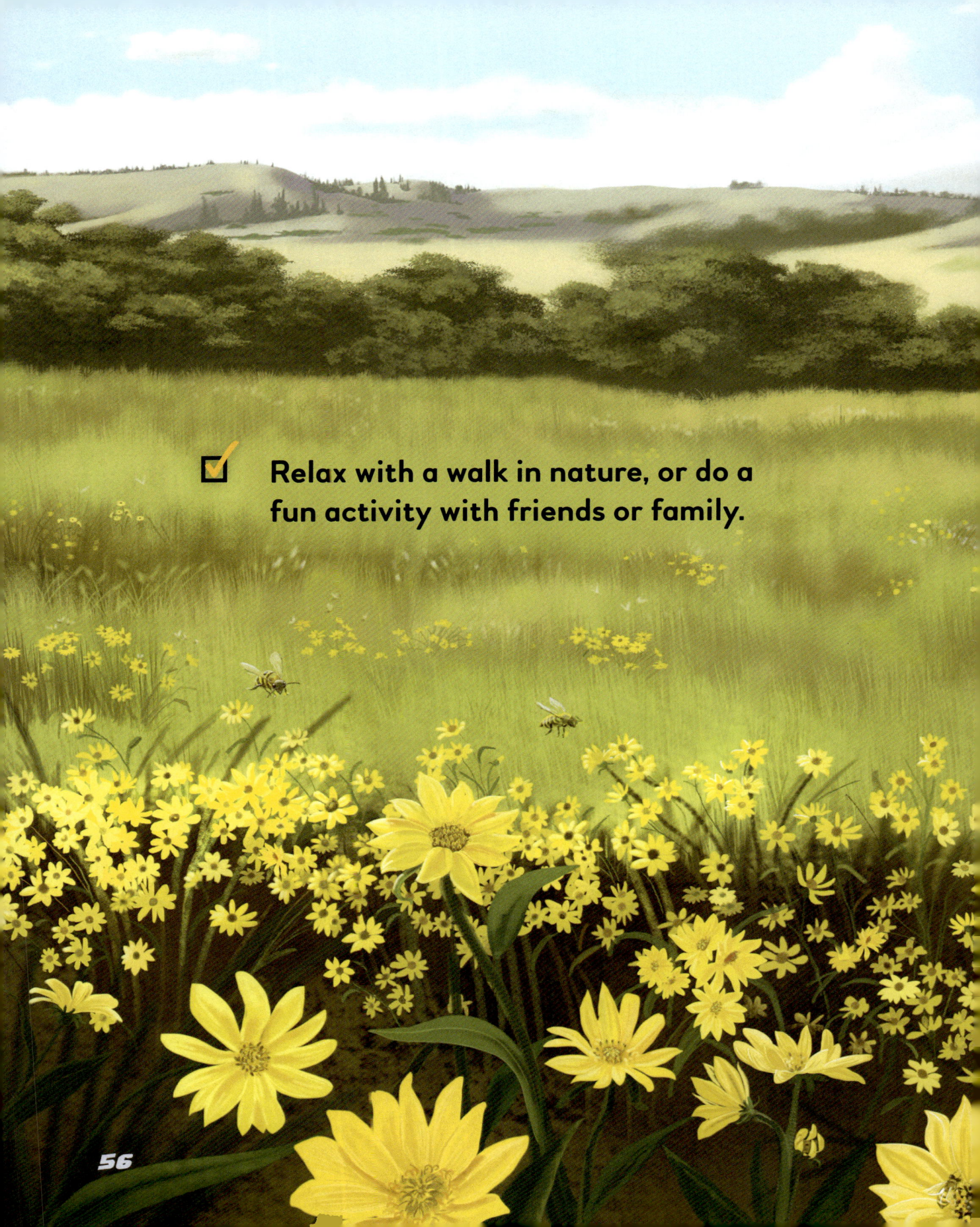

☑ **Relax with a walk in nature, or do a fun activity with friends or family.**

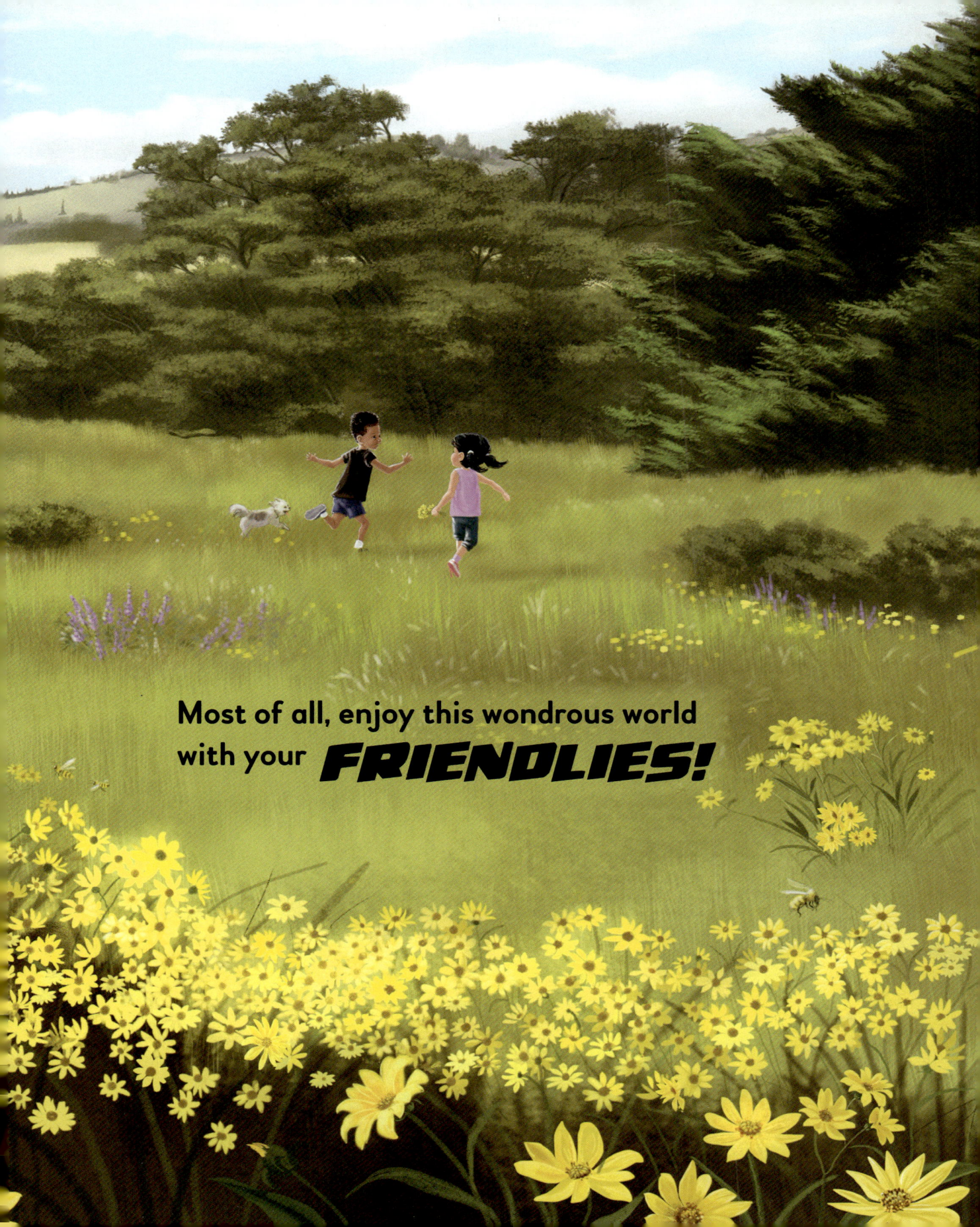
Most of all, enjoy this wondrous world with your **FRIENDLIES!**

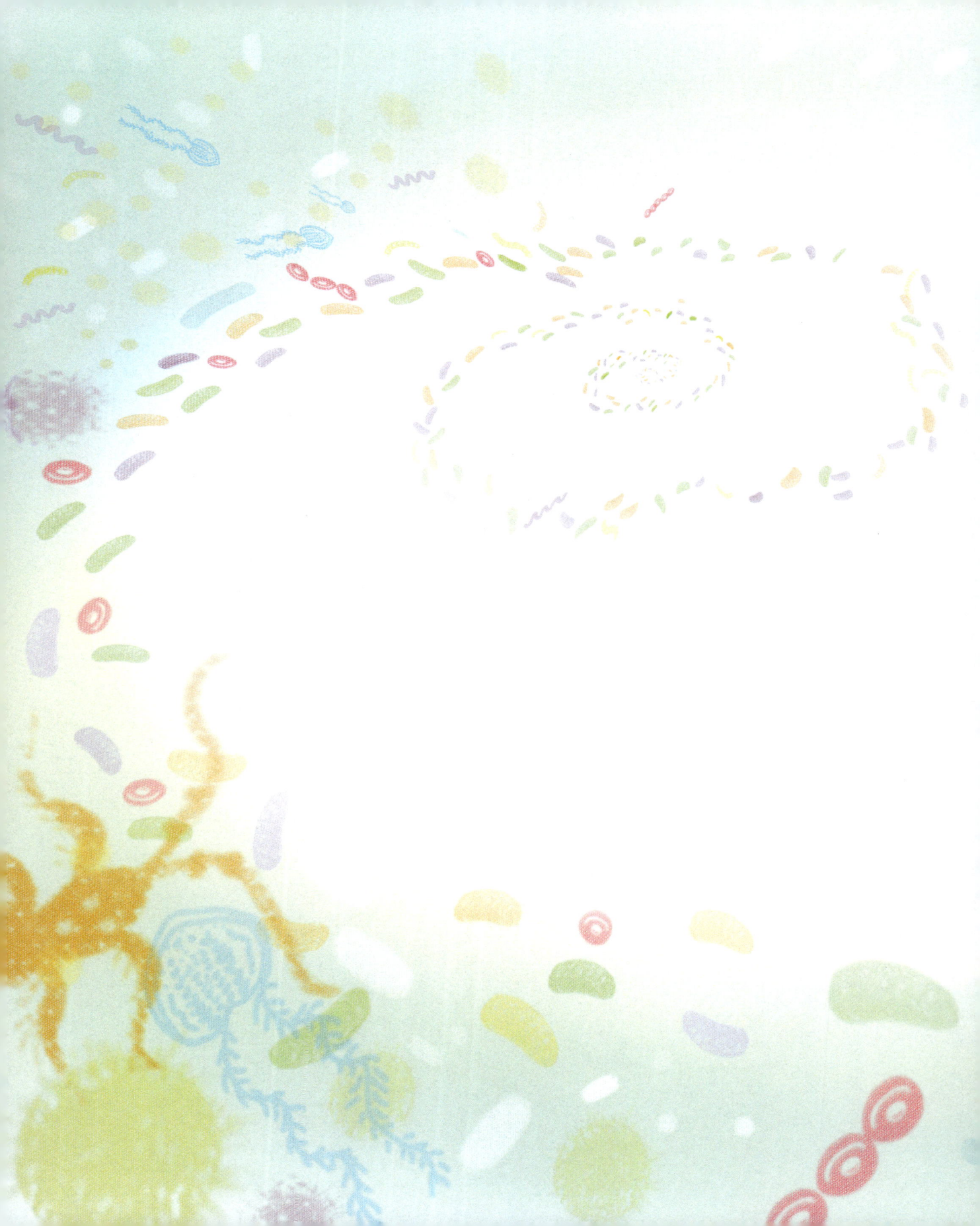

GLOSSARY

Acid (p. 16) – *a chemical compound that tastes sour.*

Alkaline (p. 30) – *a chemical compound that tastes bitter.*

Bacteria (p. 7) – *extremely tiny organisms that can only be seen under a microscope.*

Enzymes (p. 30) – *substances that speed up chemical reactions (like breaking other substances apart or joining them together)*

Fungi (p. 17) – *a type of microbe.*

Gallbladder (p. 30) – *a digestive organ that helps to digest fats.*

Germs (p. 8) – *a common name for microbes that cause disease.*

Immune system (p. 15) – *the body's defense system, protecting us from diseases caused by microbes and other invaders. The immune system is mostly made of Friendlies in the digestive tract, and includes other organs, tissues and cells of the body that work together.*

Microbes (p. 17) – *a category of organisms that includes bacteria, viruses and fungi as well as others, that can only be seen with a microscope.*

Pancreas (p. 30) – *a digestive organ that helps to digest starches and protein.*

Peristalsis (p. 33) – *a natural rhythmic squeezing that moves contents through the digestive system.*

Sebum (p. 16) – *natural oils made by glands in the skin.*

Villi (p. 30) – *microscopic finger-like folds of the inner wall of the small intestine.*

Vitamin B (p. 31) – *a group of vitamins found in foods such as grains, beans and vegetables, or made inside the body by Friendly bacteria.*

Vitamin K (p. 31) – *a vitamin found in dark leafy greens, or made inside the body by Friendly bacteria.*

ACKNOWLEDGEMENTS

I am so fortunate to be the mom of my 4 grown children Jamila, Ayanna, Jelani and Kamaria. It is a joy to see their lives unfold and witness all the creativity they each bring to the world. I am grateful to Marcia Adams Ho who brought the concepts to life with her thoughtful and beautiful illustrations, and Brett Neiman whose creative and professional design and typography was so essential in completing the book. I am thankful for Susan and Angelique of the Beverly Writers Group, who helped me to see new possibilities for the book in its early life. I am grateful for my friends Julia Schopick, author of *Honest Medicine*, and TK Mitchell, creator of Lifestyle 120 who offered support and comments. I appreciate Deanna Leah of HBG Productions for her help in expanding the reach of the book's message. Over the years I have met so many writers, friends, artists, urban farmers, nutritionists, healers, educators and community workers who have helped to shape my learning, including all my Ayurveda teachers and classmates. Notably, I thank Jacqueline Smith of Growasis, a specialist in urban gardening and homesteading, for her work in helping us cultivate a better relationship with our food and the earth and regain the homesteading skills of our ancestors. I am grateful to Dr. Kathi Kemper, who is recognized internationally as the leading authority on holistic therapies for children. My copy of her book, *The Holistic Pediatrician*, was my "dog-eared" go-to resource when I had my first practice. I am so thankful for Gary Cuneen of Seven Generations Ahead, for his ongoing work in educating and engaging the community in sustainable living. His projects include the Illinois Farm to School network, the Great Apple Crunch, and many other impactful programs. I want to especially thank my dear sisters in spirit, Suzanne and Linda, we have been on this road a very long time together! Much love to my brother David and his beautiful family. For their inspiring work in helping us understand the magnificent world of our bodies, I am grateful for the researchers of The Human Microbiome Project. As always, I honor the Ancient Ones in all cultures - upon whose shoulders we stand, such as the Hadza, one of the last hunter-gatherer tribes in Africa, whose contribution to understanding our microbiome has helped to illuminate the impact of our practices and the need for us to embrace ancient foodways.

A special message: Love you Mom, You're the best!

Philippa Norman *Author*

Dr. Philippa Norman grew up making her own herbal "medicines" in her back yard. She is an integrative physician with a focus in Ayurveda, and the author of **Three Shells for Nikki**, **Lessons From Your Body** and **Feed Your Brain: How to Boost Your Brainpower with Food**. She can be often found simmering an herbal remedy on the stove, working in her garden, playing guitar or writing.

Connect with her work at **philippanormanmd.com** and at **facebook.com/drphilippanorman**

Marcia Adams Ho *Illustrator*

Marcia graduated with a BFA from Art Center College of Design in California and began her career as a background artist in animation. She currently freelances as an illustrator specializing in book illustration and produces fine art paintings in her studio. Recent publications with Marcia's illustrations include **You Can Call Me Katelyn**, by Keri T. Collins and **The Tree Farmer's Twelve Days of Christmas**, by Aaron Burakoff. For over twenty years, Marcia gave art lessons at a local elementary school. Working with children along with raising two sons helped develop a love of using art to educate and inspire children. Marcia's illustrations capture the imagination of both children and adults alike.

Marcia also illustrated Dr. Norman's **Three Shell for Nikki**. More of Marcia's art can be viewed at **marciaadamsho.com**

Brett Neiman *Designer*

Brett has created layouts for Eve L. Ewing, Jamila Woods, José Olivarez, Camonghne Felix, Willie Perdomo, and more — and is delighted to typset and create the jacket layout for Dr. Norman's **Meet The Friendlies**.

More of Brett's work can be viewed at **brettneiman.com** Follow him **@BrettZett**